Patient Assessment and Care Planning in Nursing

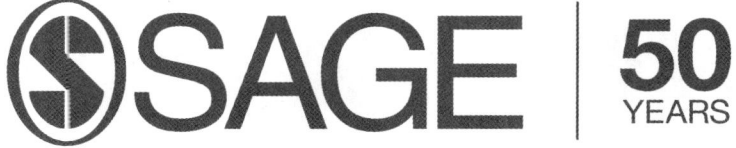

SAGE was founded in 1965 by Sara Miller McCune to support the dissemination of usable knowledge by publishing innovative and high-quality research and teaching content. Today, we publish more than 750 journals, including those of more than 300 learned societies, more than 800 new books per year, and a growing range of library products including archives, data, case studies, reports, conference highlights, and video. SAGE remains majority-owned by our founder, and after Sara's lifetime will become owned by a charitable trust that secures our continued independence.

Los Angeles | London | Washington DC | New Delhi | Singapore

Patient Assessment and Care Planning in Nursing

2nd Edition

Lioba Howatson-Jones, Mooi Standing & Susan Roberts

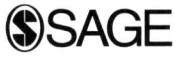
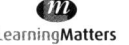

Los Angeles | London | New Delhi
Singapore | Washington DC | Boston

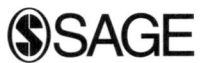 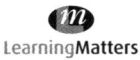

Learning Matters
An imprint of SAGE Publications Ltd
1 Oliver's Yard
55 City Road
London EC1Y 1SP

SAGE Publications Inc.
2455 Teller Road
Thousand Oaks, California 91320

SAGE Publications Ind a Pvt Ltd
B 1/I 1 Mohan Cooperative Industrial Area
Mathura Road
New Delhi 110 044

SAGE Publications Asia-Pacific Pte Ltd
3 Church Street
#10-04 Samsung Hub
Singapore 049483

Editor: Alex Clabburn
Development editor: Richenda Milton-Daws
Production controller: Chris Marke
Project management: Swales & Willis Ltd, Exeter, Devon
Marketing manager: Camille Richmond
Cover design: Wendy Scott
Typeset by: C&M Digitals (P) Ltd, Chennai, India
Printed in Great Britain by Henry Ling Limited at The Dorset Press, Dorchester, DT1 1HD

© Lioba Howatson-Jones, Mooi Standing and Susan Roberts 2012, 2015

First edition published 2012

Second edition 2015

Apart from any fair dealing for the purposes of research or private study, or criticism or review, as permitted under the Copyright, Designs and Patents Act, 1988, this publication may be reproduced, stored or transmitted in any form, or by any means, only with the prior permission in writing of the publishers, or in the case of reprographic reproduction, in accordance with the terms of licences issued by the Copyright Licensing Agency. Enquiries concerning reproduction outside those terms should be sent to the publishers.

Library of Congress Control Number: 2015930293

British Library Cataloguing in Publication data

A catalogue record for this book is available from the British Library

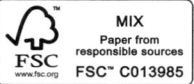

ISBN 978-1-4739-0226-8
ISBN 978-1-4739-0227-5 (pbk)

At SAGE we take sustainability seriously. Most of our products are printed in the UK using FSC papers and boards. When we print overseas we ensure sustainable papers are used as measured by the Egmont grading system. We undertake an annual audit to monitor our sustainability.

Contents

Foreword by the Series Editor, Professor Shirley Bach	ix
About the authors	xi
Acknowledgements	xiii
Introduction	1
1 Person-centred assessment and practice *Lioba Howatson-Jones*	5
2 Understanding our role in patient assessment *Lioba Howatson-Jones*	18
3 Making sense of patient information *Lioba Howatson-Jones*	33
4 Assessment tools *Lioba Howatson-Jones*	51
5 Nursing diagnosis *Lioba Howatson-Jones*	65
6 Care-planning principles *Lioba Howatson-Jones*	78
7 Relationship of nursing models to care planning *Lioba Howatson-Jones*	92
8 Ethical aspects of patient assessment dilemmas *Lioba Howatson-Jones*	108
9 Community health needs assessment *Susan Roberts*	121
10 Patient assessment and decision-making *Mooi Standing*	137
Glossary	160
References	162
Index	167

TRANSFORMING NURSING PRACTICE

Transforming Nursing Practice is a series tailor-made for pre-registration student nurses. Each book in the series is:

- Affordable
- Mapped to the NMC Standards and Essential Skills Clusters
- Full of active learning features
- Focused on applying theory to practice

Each book addresses a core topic and they have been carefully developed to be simple to use, quick to read and written in clear language.

> An invaluable series of books that explicitly relates to the NMC standards. Each book cover a different topic that students need to explore in order to develop into a qualified nurse… I would recommend this series to all Pre-Registration nursing students whatever their field or year of study.
>
> **Linda Robson**
> **Senior Lecturer, Edge Hill University**
>
> The set of books is an excellent resource for students. The series is small, easily portable and valuable. I use the whole set on a regular basis.
>
> **Fiona Davies**
> **Senior Nurse Lecturer, University of Derby**
>
> I recommend the SAGE/Learning Matters series to all my students as they are relevant and concise. Please keep up the good work.
>
> **Thomas Beary**
> **Senior Lecturer in Mental Health Nursing, University of Hertfordshire**

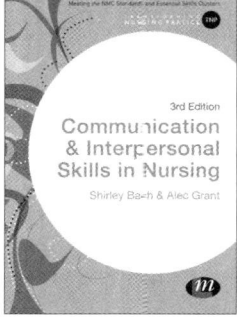
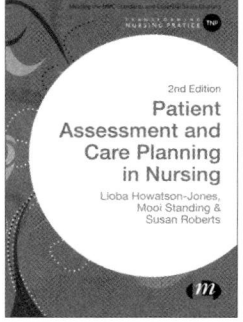
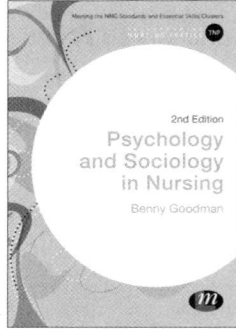

ABOUT THE SERIES EDITORS

Professor Shirley Bach is Head of the School of Health Sciences at the University of Brighton and responsible for the core knowledge titles. Previously she was head of post-graduate studies and has developed curriculum for undergraduate and pre-registration courses in a variety of subject domains.

Dr Mooi Standing is an Independent Academic Consultant (UK and International) and responsible for the personal and professional learning skills titles. She is an accredited NMC Quality Assurance Reviewer of educational programmes and a Professional Regulator Panellist on the NMC Practice Committee.

Sandra Walker is Senior Teaching Fellow in Mental Health at the University of Southampton and responsible for the mental health nursing titles. She is a Qualified Mental Health Nurse with a wide range of clinical experience spanning more than 20 years.

CORE KNOWLEDGE TITLES:
Becoming a Registered Nurse: Making the Transition to Practice
Communication and Interpersonal Skills in Nursing (3rd Ed)
Contexts of Contemporary Nursing (2nd Ed)
Getting into Nursing (2nd Ed)
Health Promotion and Public Health for Nursing Students (2nd Ed)
Introduction to Medicines Management in Nursing
Law and Professional Issues in Nursing (3rd Ed)
Leadership, Management and Team Working in Nursing (2nd Ed)
Learning Skills for Nursing Students
Medicines Management in Children's Nursing
Nursing and Collaborative Practice (2nd Ed)
Nursing and Mental Health Care
Nursing in Partnership with Patients and Carers
Passing Calculations Tests for Nursing Students (3rd Ed)
Palliative and End of Life Care in Nursing
Patient Assessment and Care Planning in Nursing (2nd Ed)
Patient and Carer Participation in Nursing
Patient Safety and Managing Risk in Nursing
Psychology and Sociology in Nursing (2nd Ed)
Successful Practice Learning for Nursing Students (2nd Ed)
Understanding Ethics in Nursing Practice
Using Health Policy in Nursing
What is Nursing? Exploring Theory and Practice (3rd Ed)

PERSONAL AND PROFESSIONAL LEARNING SKILLS TITLES:
Clinical Judgement and Decision Making for Nursing Students (2nd Ed)
Critical Thinking and Writing for Nursing Students (2nd Ed)
Evidence-based Practice in Nursing (2nd Ed)
Information Skills for Nursing Students
Reflective Practice in Nursing (2nd Ed)
Succeeding in Essays, Exams & OSCEs for Nursing Students
Succeeding in Literature Reviews and Research Project Plans for Nursing Students (2nd Ed)
Successful Professional Portfolios for Nursing Students (2nd Ed)
Understanding Research for Nursing Students (2nd Ed)

MENTAL HEALTH NURSING TITLES:
Assessment and Decision Making in Mental Health Nursing
Engagement and Therapeutic Communication in Mental Health Nursing
Medicines Management in Mental Health Nursing
Mental Health Law in Nursing
Physical Healthcare and Promotion in Mental Health Nursing
Psychosocial Interventions in Mental Health Nursing

ADULT NURSING TITLES:
Acute and Critical Care in Adult Nursing
Caring for Older People in Nursing
Medicines Management in Adult Nursing
Nursing Adults with Long Term Conditions
Safeguarding Adults in Nursing Practice
Dementia Care in Nursing

You can find more information on each of these titles and our other learning resources at **www.sagepub.co.uk**. Many of these titles are also available in various e-book formats, please visit our website for more information.

Foreword

Assessing patients' healthcare needs is not a one-off event, which involves filling in several tick boxes and a mountain of paper. It is a detailed and complex process that identifies all aspects of a patient's condition and, for those patients who are able to communicate, can be a therapeutic narrative of their personal health journey. It is also just the first step in a journey to plan nursing care using the many tools and techniques that a modern nurse has at his or her disposal.

Lioba Howatson-Jones, Mooi Standing and Susan Roberts have written a text that takes the reader from those all-important first steps through a process of systematically examining information that will lead to accurate clinical decisions, and the management of patients' care, to reach the best care outcomes. They introduce theoretical concepts and relate these to relevant case situations to hone clinical decision-making and incorporate professional values and standards. They provide a wealth of information on the tools and methods available for nurses to make decisions about patients' care and wellbeing. Importantly, the book takes a holistic approach to patient assessment and incorporates the roles of other professionals in the decisions and planning processes.

Student nurses will find this an invaluable tool in enabling them to make sense of the many aspects of assessment and decision-making and improve their confidence and knowledge. The shifting agenda to involve patients more and more in their own care is an important element of the text's approach. Finally, the text reinforces the point that assessment is a continuous process and essential to maintain high quality patient assessment and care planning.

Professor Shirley Bach
Series Editor

About the authors

Lioba Howatson-Jones is Senior Lecturer in the School of Nursing at Canterbury Christ Church University, where she teaches on pre-registration, post-registration, Master's-level courses, as well as PhD and Professional Doctoral courses. Lioba's clinical nursing background is mainly in acute nursing and practice development. She has taught at Canterbury Christ Church University since 2003 and has a particular interest in clinical supervision and person-centred care. Her research interests are in exploring nurses' learning and considering carers' needs within patient assessment. Lioba has been publishing on these and clinical topics since 1999.

Dr Mooi Standing is an independent nursing and educational consultant with over 40 years' experience including: practising mental health and adult nursing in a range of hospital and community settings; lecturing pre-registration and post-registration nursing students from certificate to Master's level and presenting scholarly papers at national nursing conferences; researching how nurses develop clinical decision-making skills and publishing articles, books and chapters on this topic for nursing students, registered nurses and advanced practitioners; and external consultancy in curriculum development and quality enhancement of nursing programmes both nationally and internationally. Mooi is also an accredited Nursing and Midwifery Council (NMC) reviewer/managing reviewer approving, monitoring and assuring the quality of nursing programmes throughout the UK.

Susan Roberts is Senior Lecturer in Adult Nursing at Canterbury Christ Church University. Her particular interests lie in the fields of tissue viability and wound care, primary care and public health, and supporting learning in practice. She is currently involved in research into wound maceration.

Acknowledgements

The authors would like to express their gratitude to their respective spouses for their support and generous 'time out' while writing this book. The continuing dedication of the Learning Matters project team in supporting and advising the authors is greatly appreciated.

In addition, Lioba Howatson-Jones would like to acknowledge the contributions of Sue West, Paul Elliott, Ann Price, Dr Chris Biela, Karen Daniels and Roger Goldsmith in the evolution of her chapters within the book.

Introduction

Who is this book for?

The new, updated edition of this book is for all student nurses who wish to develop their assessment and care planning practice and for novice practitioners who wish to extend their interrogation of practice.

What is patient assessment?

Patient assessment is a process that identifies and defines patient problems in order for solutions to be planned and implemented in line with their preferences. The purpose of this book is to introduce student nurses and other healthcare practitioners to different stages of the assessment and care planning process. It also raises some of the considerations which need to be thought about within decision-making, such as inclusion of the service user and an emphasis on person-centredness. The book takes a holistic approach to patient assessment which means that it looks at what is happening with the patient as part of a whole rather than concentrating on purely physical aspects.

The role of the nurse in assessment is changing. In order to prepare for the future you need to be ready to recognise the complexity of assessment across different settings and within changing health needs. The health agenda is shifting to involving people more in their own care. In each of the chapters you will be given opportunities for integrating your learning through the worked examples and scenarios which include assessments of people of all ages and with varying mental and physical problems. You will also be encouraged to examine the involvement of other health-care practitioners.

The structure of the book

Chapter 1 is a new chapter that sets all that follows firmly within the context of person-centred care. This chapter introduces us to the 6Cs of nursing and identifies your values and beliefs in relation to person-centred assessment and practice, before giving you some practical pointers for building upon these beliefs and putting them into action.

Chapter 2 explores the understanding of our role in patient assessment. It considers the factors that promote or inhibit effective patient assessment and looks at how to build on your current skills and knowledge of what patient assessment means. You will be asked to examine how attitudes, beliefs and stereotyping can affect the accuracy of patient assessment, and how to balance subjective and more objective forms of assessment.

Chapter 3 explores some of the different techniques needed for making sense of patient information. The chapter defines what patient information is, and identifies the roles of different

Introduction

healthcare professionals in gathering patient information. You will be encouraged to try out different questioning techniques and to differentiate between different types and forms of information and how to analyse this in order to identify nursing priorities.

Chapter 4 examines the purpose of assessment tools and looks at a range of assessment tools including the Malnutrition Universal Assessment Tool (MUST), Waterlow and the National Early Warning System (NEWS) score. You will be asked to reflect on the knowledge and skills needed to use assessment and screening tools and consider some potential problems of focusing purely on the tool. You will explore how to utilise information gained from screening and assessment to achieve a nursing diagnosis and a plan of care.

Chapter 5 defines what is meant by nursing diagnosis. It includes the history and development of nursing diagnosis, and explores how it relates to the patient assessment process. You will be asked to examine the potential benefits and problems of nursing diagnosis for the patient and healthcare professionals. You will also be encouraged to practice developing a nursing diagnosis from a patient assessment.

Chapter 6 examines why care plans are necessary and how to identify a nursing problem. You will be asked to examine the care planning stages and identify short- and long-term goals and determine interventions. You will consider examples of different care plans and be given an opportunity to develop a written care plan of your own.

Chapter 7 introduces the relevance of nursing models to the care planning process. In this chapter we will examine why models are important and look at a variety of nursing models. You will be encouraged to think about how a nursing model frames the patient assessment process and how the nursing model impacts on decision-making in care planning.

Chapter 8 introduces some of the ethical aspects of patient assessment. You will be asked to develop your understanding and application of ethical principles within patient assessment processes by reviewing ethical principles such as autonomy, beneficence, non-maleficence and justice. You will be encouraged to examine the relevance of ethical theories to patient assessment by considering some ethical dilemmas in patient assessment and resource allocation. This is followed by an exploration of some problems with ethics in theory and ethics in practice.

Chapter 9 builds on the principles covered in the previous chapters to explore the concept of the community health needs assessment with regards to identifying the causes of ill health and the desire of patients to make changes. You will be asked to examine how a community health needs assessment is a tool for promoting the health of communities and individuals and is a part of the patient assessment process. You will be encouraged to consider why the community health needs assessment is important, the steps involved in the process and application of the health needs assessment cycle.

Chapter 10 examines how patient assessment informs clinical judgement and decision-making. It relates patient assessment to Standing's (2014) ten perceptions of clinical decision-making in nursing (collaborative, observation, systematic, standardised, prioritising, experience and intuition, reflective, ethical sensitivity, accountability, and confidence), cognitive continuum theory (nine modes of practice), and newly developed 'PERSON' evaluation tool. It explores how the issues discussed in Chapters 2–9 can be addressed by applying the perceptions of decision-making and nine modes of practice to patient assessment and decision-making. The 'PERSON' evaluation tool emphasises the importance of continually reassessing and evaluating nursing decisions to ensure that they are patient-centred, promote safe and effective care, and identify areas for improvement.

The glossary at the end of the book explains specialist terms in plain English.

NMC *Standards for Pre-registration Nursing Education* and Essential Skills Clusters

The Nursing and Midwifery Council (NMC) has standards of competence which have to be met by applicants to different parts of the nursing and midwifery register. These standards are what they deem as being necessary for the delivery of safe, effective nursing and midwifery practice. This book is linked to the NMC (2010) *Standards for Pre-registration Nursing Education* which cover professional values, communication and interpersonal skills, nursing practice and decision-making and leadership, management and team working. In addition, the NMC identifies specific skills nursing students must have at various points of their training programme. These Essential Skills Clusters (ESCs) are essential abilities which students need to attain in order to practice to their full potential.

This book identifies some of the competencies and skills, within the realm of patient assessment and care planning practice, which student nurses need in order to be entered on to the NMC register. These competencies and ESCs are presented at the start of each chapter so that it is clear which of them the chapter addresses. All of the competencies and ESCs in this book relate to the *generic standards* which all nursing students must achieve.

Activities

At various stages within each chapter there are points at which you can break to undertake activities. Undertaking and understanding the activities is an important element of your understanding of the content of each chapter. You are encouraged, where appropriate, to reflect on your practice and consider how the things you have learned from working with patients might inform your understanding of patient assessment and care planning. Other activities will require you to take time away from the book to find out new information which will add to your understanding of the topic under discussion. Some activities challenge you to apply your learning to a question or scenario to help you reflect on issues and practice in more depth. A few activities

Introduction

require you to make observations during your day-to-day life or in the clinical setting. In some cases, you are encouraged to discuss your thoughts or findings with a mentor or one or more fellow students. All the activities in this book are designed to increase your understanding of the topics under discussion and how they impact upon nursing practice.

Where appropriate there are suggested or potential answers to activities at the end of the chapter. It is recommended that you try where possible to engage with the activities in order to increase your understanding of the realities of patient assessment and care planning.

Chapter 1
Person-centred assessment and practice

Lioba Howatson-Jones

> **NMC Standards for Pre-registration Nursing Education**
>
> This chapter will address the following competencies:
>
> **Domain 1: Professional values**
>
> *Competencies:*
> 1. All nurses must practise in a holistic, non-judgemental, caring and sensitive manner that avoids assumptions; supports social inclusion; recognises and respects individual choice; and acknowledges diversity. Where necessary, they must challenge inequality, discrimination and exclusion from access to care.
>
> **Domain 2: Communication and interpersonal skills**
>
> *Competencies:*
> 2. All nurses must use a range of communication skills and technologies to support person-centred care and enhance quality and safety. They must ensure people receive all the information they need in a language and manner that allows them to make informed choices and share decision-making. They must recognise when language interpretation or other communication support is needed and know how to obtain it.
> 3. All nurses must use the full range of communication methods, including verbal, non-verbal and written, to acquire, interpret and record their knowledge and gain an understanding of people's needs. They must be aware of their own values and beliefs and the impact this may have on their communication with others. They must take account of the many different ways in which people communicate and how these may be influenced by ill health, disability and other factors, and be able to recognise and respond effectively when a person finds it hard to communicate.

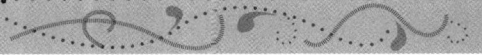

NMC Essential Skills Clusters

This chapter will address the following ESCs:

Cluster: Care, compassion and communication
2. People can trust the newly registered graduate nurse to engage in person-centred care, empowering people to make choices about how their needs are met when they are unable to meet them for themselves.

By the first progression point:
1. Takes a person-centred, personalised approach to care.

By the second progression point:
2. Actively empowers people to be involved in the assessment and care planning process.

Chapter aims

After reading this chapter, you will be able to:

- identify your values and beliefs in relation to person-centred assessment and practice;
- assess how you can contribute to working in ways that are person-centred;
- discuss the 6Cs and how they relate to person-centred practice;
- identify workplace cultures that are not working in person-centred ways;
- develop strategies for dealing with practice which is not person-centred and using the 6Cs.

Case study: Sonia's experience of someone with learning difficulties

Sonia was a midwifery student completing a placement in a high risk birthing centre in her second year. Her supervisor Breed was a highly experienced midwife. Sonia still had a number of objectives to achieve in order to progress to the third year including empowering diverse service users, and she discussed this with Breed as part of her learning contract discussion. The phone interrupted their discussion and Breed took details. When Breed had finished the conversation she informed Sonia that a woman called Mandy was coming by ambulance with a difficult birth presentation, and that she had learning difficulties.

Sonia was concerned about how she would communicate with Mandy as she had no experience of dealing with people with learning difficulties. She imagined that Mandy would be terrified with no idea about what was happening to her. Sonia also imagined that Mandy would probably have difficulty processing detailed information.

Mandy arrived with her mother Ruby who was looking distressed. Sonia immediately went to reassure Ruby that they would help Mandy as quickly as possible, while Breed got ready to examine Mandy. Breed ascertained that Mandy's baby was a shoulder presentation requiring a caesarean delivery and contacted the

> *obstetrician and anaesthetist immediately. Throughout this Mandy was crying in pain and Sonia tried to help calm her, but Mandy was getting cross. Sonia tried to explain what they were doing, but realised that she was using medical terms and Mandy did not understand. She felt helpless, but persevered by asking Mandy to tell her what she was experiencing. The obstetrician arrived, completed her assessment and explained the process for proceeding to caesarean to Ruby and asked her to sign the consent. Sonia observed how Ruby explained to Mandy what was happening, before going with her to theatre. Mandy's baby was a large baby boy whom she named Liam.*
>
> *Afterwards, when taking a break in the coffee room Sonia listened to the midwives discussing Mandy's case. A number wondered how Mandy would cope with a baby. One midwife called Smini said that it was not fair on the baby. Others argued that Mandy had the support of her mother and that some women were not as fortunate as that. Sonia found herself thinking that Mandy would need a lot of support because of her learning difficulties.*

Introduction

Working in person-centred ways has become a key focus for quality improvement of health and social care following recent highly publicised deficits in care provision in services across the United Kingdom (UK). As is highlighted in the case study above, some staff still hold values and beliefs which are not person-centred and which are likely to influence the way they practice. This chapter will begin by providing some of the background to the Quality Improvement Agenda in the UK and then proceed to identifying some definitions of what person-centredness is, and why it is so important. The chapter will outline the importance of developing self-awareness of our own values and beliefs and how these contribute to workplace culture. The chapter will conclude with some strategies on how you can develop working in person-centred ways that also encompass the '6Cs'.

Background to Quality Improvement in Health and Social Care in the UK

Deficits in care and compassion have recently been identified in a number of high profile reports about failures to provide the requisite level of care to patients and/or service users in a number of health and social care organisations (Equality and Human Rights Commission, 2011; Francis, 2013; Keogh, 2013). These issues are not confined to England, but appear in the rest of the UK as well, although are often explained as isolated incidents (Andrews and Butler, 2014) despite statistics for healthcare complaints rising sharply (Northern Ireland Ombudsman, 2013; SPSO, 2014). Indeed, healthcare failures were identified as a worldwide problem ten years ago (Walshe and Shortall, 2004) and again more recently (New South Wales Department of Health, 2009). However, what appears to have changed is the focus which has moved to examining organisational and interpersonal cultures and how these can influence people's behaviours. Against this background of negative rhetoric one has to ask the question: 'What is going wrong with caring?'

This question can also be more specifically directed towards nursing which is singled out as a problem in many of the care failure reports. One response has come from the Chief Nurse for England Jane Cummins who, with the Department for Health (GB) in 2012, developed a vision of compassion in practice for nursing, midwifery and care staff. This is to be rolled out to all health service staff from 2014 by NHS England (Stephenson, 2014). This vision sets out the core values which need to underpin practice which are commonly known as the '6Cs'. They are:

Care

Care is our core business and that of our organisations, and the care we deliver helps the individual person and improves the health of the whole community. Caring defines us and our work. People receiving care expect it to be right for them, consistently, throughout every stage of their life

Compassion

Compassion is how care is given through relationships based on empathy, respect and dignity – it can also be described as intelligent kindness, and is central to how people perceive their care.

Competence

Competence means all those in caring roles must have the ability to understand an individual's health and social needs and the expertise, clinical and technical knowledge to deliver effective care and treatments based on research and evidence.

Communication

Communication is central to successful caring relationships and to effective team working.

Listening is as important as what we say and do, and essential for 'No decision about me without me'. Communication is the key to a good workplace with benefits for those in our care and staff alike.

Courage

Courage enables us to do the right thing for the people we care for, to speak up when we have concerns and to have the personal strength and vision to innovate and to embrace new ways of working.

Commitment

A commitment to our patients and populations is a cornerstone of what we do. We need to build on our commitment to improve the care and experience of our patients, to take action to make this vision and strategy a reality for all and meet the health, care and support challenges ahead.

(Department of Health and NHS Commissioning Board, 2012, p13)

What this means in practice is treating people we care for in a kindly way with dignity and respect, listening to their wishes and speaking up for them when required. This requires confidence in ourselves, our profession and in each other to do the right thing. Blaming a lack of time or resources is not an option for poor practice. Throughout the chapters in this book you will be asked to review some of the scenarios to identify which of the '6Cs' are most applicable to the case. In this way you will be able to become familiar with interpreting how the '6Cs' play out in practice.

While a lack of resources and leadership and rising workload are very real issues for health and social care organisations, there appears to be a fundamental shift within some individuals who are employed by them, which apparently leads to uncaring attitudes and behaviours – some might call this compassion fatigue where the ability to cope becomes overwhelmed (Figley, 1995). The Francis Report (2013) specifically calls for improvement in care and compassion and greater emphasis on involving people in our care. Similarly, Scotland is focusing their healthcare improvement work on collaborating with people, their families and carers, bringing people together through, for example, the Person-Centred Health and Care Collaborative (2014). Similar ventures are in their infancy in Northern Ireland and Wales. However, it is encouraging that lessons appear to be being learned from the seismic Francis (2013) report through a change in emphasis from competency to the inclusion of caring attitudes and behaviours in quality audits. You are encouraged to complete Activity 1.1 to consider a different perspective.

Activity 1.1 — Reflection

Watch the video clip which can be found at: **www.youtube.com/watch?v=XOCda6OiYpg**

How would you want to respond to the quality concerns raised previously?

There are some outline suggestions at the end of the chapter.

Within your answer to the activity you might have considered your professional values and what your profession does well, and how you want to portray this to others. We move on now to consider what person-centredness is.

What is person-centredness?

In order to define person-centredness we need to first consider, 'What is a person?' Some define personhood as grounded in feelings of being in the world (Heron, 1992), while others suggest that such a being has rational capability and basic moral status or human rights (Ikäheimo and Laitinen, 2007), or more broadly possesses attributes that make them a person (Dewing, 2008). Carl Rogers, a well known psychologist and humanist, argues that person-centredness is a way of being that sees the whole person embedded in their lifeworld (Rogers, 1995). What this means is that we need to recognise that people do not exist on their own, but are connected to others and to important events and interests in their lives that make them who they are. Building therapeutic relationships with people uses values of respect, empathy, empowerment and being genuine. You might like to complete Activity 1.2 to consider what makes you the person you are.

> **Activity 1.2** — *Reflection*
>
> Consider the following:
>
> - Who are the people you are connected with?
> - What are the significant events in your life?
> - What is important to you?
>
> Based on your answers above what kind of person do you consider yourself to be?
>
> *As this activity is based on your personal experience there is no outline answer at the end of the chapter.*

Consequently, if our ideas about what a person is are connected to how we interact with 'persons' in the world, what does being person-centred mean? Person-centredness has long been debated in the literature and often been used interchangeably with similar terms such as patient-centredness which confuses the issue. Some definitions of person-centredness and person-centred care can be found in Box 1.1.

Person-centredness	*A standing or status that is bestowed upon one human by others, in the context of relationship and social being. It implies recognition, respect and trust.* (Kitwood, 1997, p8)
	Person-centredness is an approach to practice established through the formation and fostering of healthful relationships between all care providers, older people and others significant to them in their lives. It is underpinned by values of respect for persons, individual right to self-determination, mutual respect and understanding. It is enabled by cultures of empowerment that foster continuous approaches to practice development. (McCormack et al., 2013, p193)
Person-centred care	*Care that: is focused on clients/users; promotes independence and autonomy rather than control; involves services that are reliable and flexible and chosen by users; and tends to be offered by those working in a collaborative/team philosophy.* (Innes et al., 2006, pix)

	… four different perspectives each of which … ultimately shapes the way person-centredness is operationalised in practice – an attributes perspective, a reflective perspective, a moral perspective and an embodied perspective. (McCormack and McCance, 2010, p5)

Box 1.1: Definitions of person-centredness and person-centred care

What these definitions have in common is respect, trust and a right to self-determination. This can be enabled by practice development activity, which explores ways of working differently and critically reflects on how you are involved in your practice and with your patient. Often the starting point is an analysis of the language used to describe your practice and your patient/service user. This can reflect your values and beliefs about person-centredness which is what we move on to consider now.

Identifying values and beliefs

You will have developed your own values and beliefs through your upbringing, life experiences and people you interact with. Identifying your own values and beliefs is an important starting point for self-awareness. To do this you first need to be clear what a value is and what a belief is. Some consider values to represent the authentic self in terms of identity behaviours (Stets and Carter, 2011) while others suggest that values can shift over time (Morris, 2012). Beliefs on the other hand are our convictions about the way we see things regardless of evidence. Through making explicit our values and beliefs we are taking the first steps to making them a reality in our work, practice and workplace. A match between what we say we believe and what we do is one of the hallmarks of effective individuals, teams and organisations (Manley, 2000).

Activity 1.3 — Critical thinking

You are now invited to complete a values clarification exercise to explore your values and beliefs about person-centredness. This may take you approximately 30 minutes. A values clarification exercise is a grand title for a simple exercise designed to access and clarify the values and beliefs we hold about something. For the purpose of developing an understanding of person-centredness you are being asked to consider the following statements:

- I believe the ultimate purpose of person-centredness is ……….
- I believe this purpose can be achieved by ……….
- I believe the factors that inhibit or enable this purpose to be achieved include ……….
- Other values/beliefs that I hold about person-centredness are ……….

Chapter 1
continued ...

> You might like to list three or four fundamental values which underpin your beliefs and which guide your actions and behaviours. Once you have completed the exercise make a note of any questions you are asking yourself. This exercise is adapted from Manley (2003).
>
> *As this activity is based on your personal ideas there is no outline answer at the end of the chapter.*

It is important to understand our own values and beliefs because when we meet people who are different from us it can be easy to fill in gaps in our understanding with our own values and beliefs rather than finding out what their values and beliefs are. The same applies to the variety of people we work with. Recognising and valuing someone elses's perspective is a key aspect of being person-centred, and of starting to understand different cultures. We move forward now to consider workplace culture.

Workplace culture

Culture is experienced as a social phenomenon involving people in different ways. Manley et al. state that workplace culture is:

> *The most immediate culture experienced and/or perceived by staff, patients, users and other key stakeholders. This is the culture that impacts directly on the delivery of care. It both influences and is influenced by the organisation and corporate cultures with which it interfaces as well as other idiocultures through staff relationships and movement.*
> (Manley et al., 2011, p4)

Idiocultures are the behaviours and knowledge which a group of people hold and with which they interact. A group that work together may have settled into a particular way of thinking and behaving, which they do unconsciously, and into which they socialise new members. For example, the case study at the start of this chapter hints at the kind of workplace culture in which some midwives exist. Some of these hints (such as assumptions about people with learning difficulties through questioning Mandy's ability to cope) appear in the discussion in the coffee room after Mandy has given birth to Liam. You are invited to think more deeply about culture and what culture means to you through Activity 1.4.

Activity 1.4 — *Critical thinking*

> Begin this activity by thinking about what the word 'culture' means to you. A useful way to creatively think about this can be to take a walk and look at nature around you; how different things are ordered, how they perhaps grow co-operatively or not, what is successful and what is not. Try to look critically and notice details in a mindful way (see Glossary) that helps you to conceptualise what culture might be. Mindful means becoming aware of things which we normally take for granted. When you have noted down the points you think are important enter the word 'culture' into Google and consider the results. How do these compare and contrast to

your ideas? Now, think about how culture is formed and what you think (from your experience) makes it good or bad. List the attributes of both.

There is an outline answer at the end of the chapter.

You might have thought about a workplace where you felt everyone worked really well together or one where there was tension and disagreement. The important thing is to be able to critically analyse the elements of each so that you can recognise what the attributes are. Consider the following case study and answer the questions at the end to help develop your thinking.

Case study: Rob's observation of workplace culture

Rob was a radiography student completing a sampling placement on a care of the older person ward. He was only there for a week. His collaborative practice module in university had covered some theory relating to workplace culture and for his assignment he needed to observe a workplace culture which was different from his own. Rob thought that this sampling placement would provide him with a good opportunity to observe the workplace culture in this area. He discussed this with the ward manager, Martin, who was keen to hear about his observations as he was trying to make some changes.

On his first day Rob was welcomed by Eileen, an older nurse who was approaching retirement. She spoke about this often. She said she loved the job, but it was getting harder with all the changes and new technology. After showing Rob round, Eileen introduced him to other members of the team. She also introduced him to some of the patients she seemed particularly fond of. However, Rob noted the contrast when a member of staff from another ward came to ask about borrowing something. Eileen was quite sharp in her response. The same happened when one of the kitchen staff came to say that a patient had spilled water on the floor.

Rob observed that the ward smelt fresh and was reasonably tidy. The clinical room seemed almost regimented in its order. He was assigned to accompany a healthcare assistant called Judith while she completed patient vital sign observations. He noted that she wheeled the observation machine from patient to patient and that she called them all 'duck' while explaining what she was doing. Other staff did not appear concerned about this and the patients appeared to respond positively.

During coffee break Rob listened to the conversation in the staff room. It was mostly about what people were planning to do at the weekend or on future holidays. However, one part of dialogue caught his attention when Eileen started to talk about the changes Martin was making to the ward. Although Eileen could see the need for progress she felt that 'old timers' like herself were not consulted, despite their years of experience. Eileen looked around the staff room for support, and May, a nurse who usually worked nights, started to snipe about Martin. Rob decided to leave the room at this point.

At lunchtime Rob observed the handover. There was some chat at the start about unrelated issues and then the relevant nurses handed over their patients. Rob noticed that the language used was very medically

> orientated with little comment on how people might be feeling. The handover was predominantly about the tasks which had been fulfilled.
>
> Rob made a few notes about his observations to help with his assignment preparation. What was of greater concern to him at present was how he was going to feed back his observations to Martin as he did not want to appear to have been 'spying'.
>
> 1. What observations do you think Rob is likely to have made about this ward culture?
> 2. In what way is Rob feeling uncomfortable about providing Martin with feedback?
> 3. How might Rob present his feedback?
>
> There are some outline answers at the end of the chapter.

What the case study shows is that workplace culture is something which can cause you to respond in ways which are contrary to your values and beliefs as other factors come into play such as power and authority. It also shows that workplace culture is dynamic and not fixed and therefore can be changed by the participants. Therefore, if you are thinking and working in person-centred ways, you can make a positive contribution to your workplace culture. We move forward now to consider how you can work in ways that are person-centred.

Person-centred ways of working

Being person-centred in our working means first of all developing person-centred thinking in the way we communicate with others and how we frame our practice. This can be difficult when healthcare systems appear to be committed to standardising practice, reducing the opportunities for getting to know patients as people (McCormack et al., 2013). You need to be prepared to use the time you have to attentively listen to what people are saying – whether patient or staff member – and develop empowering ways of problem-solving that support positive ways of working. Attentive listening involves the following:

- a facilitative attitude which shows trust in the person's potential;
- attending, observing and listening, showing you're 'being with' someone – this might be called sympathetic presence;
- processing what you have heard by thoughtfully searching for meaning;
- being aware of your internal dialogue, checking for potential actions or assumptive obstacles.

(Egan, 2014)

Doing this requires you to focus on finding solutions with people rather than dwelling on problems which maybe they can do nothing about. Being solution-focused means interpreting things differently with an emphasis on positive elements such as the strengths and resources that people bring from their lives to achieve their goals (Lynch et al., 2008). The person, not the problem, is at the centre of enquiry. The person's ideas, language and expertise are privileged, and the way of being with persons is proactive rather than reactive (MacAllister, 2007). For this type of thinking you need to use imagination and creativity as well as reasoning. Their motivation is likely to increase because you are building on people's strengths, as you generate personal plans. In this way both the person and the health professional take responsibility to try creative solutions. Consider the following case study and then answer the questions at the end in order to help you develop some person-centred practice solutions.

Case study: Harriet's hair solution

Harriet is a mental health nurse working in a unit with older persons, many of whom have dementia. Last week she admitted a new lady called June. June had been living alone, with neighbours doing what they could to help her as she had no living family. However, when she arrived she appeared very unkempt with extremely knotted hair and stained clothing. Harriet had gently settled June in to the unit with a hot drink, and gave her options for what she wanted to do. It was clear that June was disorientated.

This week June has appeared more settled until anyone tries to go near brushing her hair, when she starts to scream and becomes very agitated. Harriet sits down with June and asks her whether she liked going to the hairdresser. June starts to talk about when she was a teenager with a beehive hairdo getting admiring looks from the boys. Her hair was her pride and joy until there was a house fire at home and she was seriously injured. She remembered how horrible she looked with burned hair. It took months for her hair to grow back. She doesn't like people touching it!

Harriet asked June if she had any photos of her beehive hair. June said she had a small one in her bag. Harriet looked at it with June. She said she knew a lady called Maureen who was really good at doing hair and asked June if she wanted to meet her. June mumbled maybe. Harriet arranged for Maureen to come in at the end of the week and asked Maureen to first show June what she could do by working on Harriet's hair. She noted a spark of interest from June when Maureen started working on Harriet's hair. When Maureen had finished Harriet asked June if she wanted Maureen to help her with her hair and what she wanted doing? June responded positively and Maureen was able to gently release the tangles from June's hair and create a lovely style for her. Harriet and June compared their styles at the end and had a good laugh together.

QUESTIONS

1. How does Harriet's care plan compare or contrast with what we have discussed in this chapter?
2. How does Harriet's care plan compare to what you would do?
3. How can you develop imaginative thinking about finding solutions with persons?

There is an outline answer at the end of this chapter.

Activity 1.5 *Critical thinking*

Look back at the '6Cs' and then at case studies/scenarios in this chapter. Can you identify which of the '6Cs' are actively evident in the scenario?

There is an outline answer at the end of the chapter.

Chapter summary

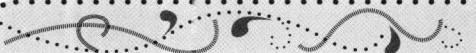

This chapter has explored the concepts of the '6Cs' and person-centredness with regards to values and beliefs, workplace culture and explored more positive ways of working with people that encourage motivation and collaboration. Through the activities you have been given opportunities to identify your own values and beliefs and definitions of culture, in order to help you understand how you can develop your person-centred practice further.

Activities: brief outline answers

Activity 1.1 Reflection [page 9]

You might have considered how your profession exhibits care and compassion and respects patients/clients/service users with some specific examples. You might also have thought about writing your own poem or narrative to show this.

Activity 1.4 Critical thinking [page 12]

You might have thought that culture meant a shared set of behaviours or seeing things in similar ways to others. When Googling the word 'culture', you might have discovered diverse meanings such as a group of people sharing certain characteristics; acting on certain assumptions; that culture exists on different levels. Your list of attributes for good cultures might have included self-awareness, clarity of roles and priorities, insight into the consequences of actions, giving and receiving effective feedback, high challenge and high support, teamwork and open communication. Your list of attributes for a bad culture might have identified working individually, lack of clarity of roles, unclear priorities, closed communication, little or no feedback, and high challenge with low support.

Case study: Rob's observation of workplace culture [page 13]

Rob is likely to have observed the inconsistent welcome given to different people which is likely to have influenced how they responded, felt, thought and behaved. He is also likely to have observed the use of non-person-centred language to patients and staff and the task-based approach to care and talking about care. This reveals that regardless of what the ward philosophy might be, the care experienced by patients and staff is not person-centred. Rob is likely to feel uncomfortable because he feels some of the socialisation effects from the conversation in the staff room, and he now has to show that he does not want to be socialised to think as the group do. On the other hand, he also does not want to be socialised into Martin's way of working either. Rob is likely to feel uncomfortable because he does not see himself as belonging to either group. Providing feedback will make him feel that he is not being authentic. Rob might present his feedback as the observations of an outsider. In this way he might align himself to a more neutral patient role.

Case study: Harriet's hair solution [page 15]

Harriet's care plan is based on getting to know June as a person through talking about areas of her life that she is able to remember. We don't know what the culture on the unit is, or what Harriet's values are specifically, but the fact that she is willing to take time to get to know June suggests that it might be supportive to working in person-centred ways and that Harriet's values are about respecting persons. You might be more used to task-based care plans which are mainly physically focused, or you may be very familiar with working out solutions with people. The way to develop imaginative thinking is to take a risk as Harriet did when asking June about her previous hairdresser experience. Through such gentle probing solutions may start to emerge in creative ways.

Activity 1.5 Critical thinking [page 16]

The first case study involving Sonia and Mandy demonstrates use of care and communication. The case study involving Rob shows commitment and courage. The case study involving Harriet and June demonstrates commitment, compassion and courage to innovate.

Further reading

Francis, R (2013) *Report of the Mid Staffordshire NHS Foundation Trust Public Inquiry: Executive Summary.* London: HMSO. Available at **www.midstaffspublicinquiry.com**, accessed January 2015.

Keogh, B (2013) Review into the quality of care and treatment provided by 14 hospital trusts in England: overview report. Available at **www.nhs.uk/NHSEngland/bruce-keogh-review/Documents/outcomes/keogh-review-final-report.pdf**, accessed January 2015.

Kitwood, T (1997) *Dementia Reconsidered: The Person Comes First.* Milton Keynes: Open University Press.

Manley, K, Sanders, K, Cardiff, S and Webster, J (2011) Effective workplace culture: the attributes, enabling factors and consequences of a new concept. *International Practice Development Journal,* 1 (2) Article 1. Available at **www.fons.org/library/journal/volume1-issue2/article1**, accessed January 2015.

Useful websites

www.bapca.org.uk

Although this website is predominantly aimed at counsellors, nevertheless it has some useful reading around the work of Carl Rogers and a person-centred approach, and will also be helpful to those working in other fields, particularly mental health.

www.helensandersonassociates.co.uk/reading-room/how/person-centred-thinking.aspx

This website offers a variety of resources and examples of person-centred practice with different groups of people including child, adult and mental health nurses.

www.health.org.uk/areas-of-work/topics/person-centred-care

This website offers a number of exemplars and resources which can be used to aid person-centred decision-making.

Chapter 2
Understanding our role in patient assessment

Lioba Howatson-Jones

NMC Standards for Pre-registration Nursing Education

This chapter will address the following competencies:

Domain 1: Professional values
2. All nurses must practise in a holistic, non-judgemental, caring and sensitive manner that avoids assumptions; supports social inclusion; recognises and respects individual choice; and acknowledges diversity. Where necessary, they must challenge inequality, discrimination and exclusion from access to care.

Domain 3: Nursing practice and decision-making
3. All nurses must carry out comprehensive, systematic nursing assessments that take account of relevant physical, social, cultural, psychological, spiritual, genetic and environmental factors, in partnership with service users and others through interaction, observation and measurement.

Domain 4: Leadership, management and team working
4. All nurses must be self-aware and recognise how their own values, principles and assumptions may affect their practice. They must maintain their own personal and professional development, learning from experience, through supervision, feedback, reflection and evaluation.

NMC Essential Skills Clusters

This chapter will address the following ESCs:

Cluster: Care, compassion and communication
2. People can trust the newly registered graduate nurse to engage in person-centred care empowering people to make choices about how their needs are met when they are unable to meet them for themselves.

By the first progression point:
1. Takes a person-centred, personalised approach to care.

By the second progression point:
2. Actively empowers people to be involved in the assessment and care-planning process.
3. People can trust the newly registered graduate nurse to respect them as individuals and strive to help them preserve their dignity at all times.

By the first progression point:
1. Demonstrates respect for diversity and individual preference, valuing differences, regardless of personal view.
2. Engages with people in a way that ensures dignity is maintained through making appropriate use of the environment, self and skills and adopting an appropriate attitude.

Chapter aims

After reading this chapter you should be able to:

- identify what the nurse's role is in patient assessment and why it is so important;
- consider four ways of knowing and the nature of truth;
- use Standing's cognitive continuum and identify its relevance to nurses and patient assessment;
- understand some consequences of stereotyping.

Introduction

Scenario: Mr Tyler's dog bite

Mr Tyler keeps a number of very large dogs. One of them recently bit him on the left hand while he was trying to separate a dog fight in his back garden. Mr Tyler attended the local minor injuries unit where he had the wound cleaned and dressed and was given a tetanus booster and a course of antibiotics.

You are on placement with the community district nurses, who have been asked to check the wound and continue the dressings as necessary. Mr Tyler answers the door and you are faced by a man who has numerous piercings and tattoos and who is wearing a death metal T-shirt. You feel quite intimidated. Before you can clean the wound, the old dressing has to be removed and it appears quite dirty. The district nurse asks Mr Tyler what he has been doing to get the wound dressing so dirty. Mr Tyler starts to get angry. The district nurse tries to calm him by saying that until she knows what his needs are she

Chapter 2

continued ...

> *cannot offer any potential solutions to keep the wound clean. Mr Tyler identifies that he repairs motorbikes and needs to use both hands to do this and cannot take time off as he has a number of projects due for completion. The district nurse suggests that he could wear gloves while he does this and identifies where he might buy these. She also emphasises the importance of keeping the wound clean in order to facilitate healing. She explains that the healing process will take longer because Mr Tyler is still using his hand. Afterwards you ask if she felt intimidated. The district nurse explains the importance of meeting people where they are. Her priority is assessing the patient's needs rather than imposing an ideal solution.*

The case study above highlights the importance of courage – one of the 6Cs – as you confront your fear and focus on the person instead (to review the 6Cs, see Chapter 1). In the last chapter you were asked to explore your values and beliefs around person-centredness. Our values can also form part of the frame for patient assessment. The Nursing and Midwifery Council (NMC) (2008, 2015) code of conduct clearly states the values nurses are expected to use within their professional work. Nurses come from different cultural contexts and backgrounds, where their own individual value systems will have started to develop. It is important to recognise the origins of your attitudes and beliefs and how they might influence your patient assessments, in order to identify what is appropriate and necessary when assessing a patient. The case study above highlights how someone's dress and personal presentation can be interpreted as reflecting values and beliefs that are very different from yours, and you may find this challenging and potentially intimidating. How you feel can influence the way you frame your patient assessment and may also affect how much time it takes. It is important, as the case study identifies, to work with the patient in planning the patient's care. This chapter will explore factors that may promote or inhibit effective patient assessment. It will also look at how to build on your current skills and knowledge to develop your patient assessment technique. It will begin by clarifying what patient assessment means and then continue by considering how attitudes, beliefs and stereotyping can affect the accuracy of patient assessment, and how to balance subjective and objective forms of assessment.

What is patient assessment?

Patient assessment is a process of evaluating the patient's mental, physical, social, cultural, spiritual and personal needs and of identifying the patient's wishes in relation to the options available. Failure to recognise and respond to patient needs can result in those needs not being met and in a failure of care (Barrett et al., 2009; McCormack and McCance, 2010). This will be detrimental to the patient and may be professionally damaging for health professionals caring for the patient, including you. For example, you may not pass the practice assessment component of your programme. Within patient assessment, it is important to consider the patient's lifeworld in order to identify that patient's needs. 'Lifeworld' refers to the history, culture, people, relationships and situations which are part of a patient's experience (West et al., 2007). The following case study helps to illustrate these points.

Case study: Graham's medical ward placement

Graham was in the second year of his nurse preparation programme, working on a ward specialising in diabetes care. Aaron, a student undertaking a law degree, was a newly diagnosed diabetic struggling with managing his diabetes and sugar level control. Graham was asked by his mentor Brett to complete Aaron's admission assessment.

Graham checked Aaron's notes before meeting him and identified that he had had two hypoglycaemic episodes in the last few days, the most recent being one which brought him to accident and emergency.

Graham asked Aaron about his medical history and then checked his understanding of diabetes. He noted that Aaron was a strict orthodox Jew and that he had been given advice from the dietician previously. Graham assumed that Aaron would therefore know what foods he could have and those he needed to take care with. Aaron told Graham that he had completed his exams recently which he thought might have contributed to his hypoglycaemic episodes due to the stress affecting his eating pattern.

Graham completed the assessment documenting Aaron's religion in the biographical section. He was pleased with managing to complete the paperwork and informed Brett that Aaron's admission was complete without highlighting the issues about Aaron's recent stress and disruption to his eating pattern.

Activity 2.1   Critical thinking

In the case study above, what might be the repercussions for Graham, Brett and Aaron of failing to report the issue of Aaron's stress and disrupted eating in the patient assessment? How does this scenario relate to the 6Cs?

An outline answer is given at the end of the chapter.

As the case study highlights, assessment undertaken with rather than on patients is preferable because an inclusive approach is more likely to gain patient co-operation and more accurate information. Such an assessment is called 'person-centred' because not only does it take account of the patient's wishes, but it also takes account of the patient's lifeworld. This means all the elements that make up the patient's everyday life, including relevant family/friends, daily activities, preferences and interests. As the case study highlights, adding the information about Aaron's recent stress and eating pattern enables a broader assessment of his needs, and more focused use of resources. The purpose of assessment is to identify what treatment, services or care the patient needs but, more importantly, whether the patient also wants them (Field and Smith, 2008, p18). Graham's response suggests he is focused on the task of admitting Aaron and completing the documentation rather than listening attentively to what Aaron is saying. We now proceed to look at the nurse's role in patient assessment.

Chapter 2

What is the nurse's role in patient assessment?

Patient assessment draws on a variety of knowledge. Carper (1978) previously defined the variety of knowledge required in nursing as *empirics, aesthetics and ethics* (Carper, 1978, p14). In essence, what this means is that evidence-based knowledge should be used to underpin patient assessment as a systematic process, but that employing caring behaviours to help build a therapeutic relationship with your patient is of equal importance and also needs to be sustained by ethical behaviour. The Royal College of Nursing (2003) has acknowledged that trying to define the knowledge that nurses use is complex and not necessarily helpful, as nursing is constantly evolving. More recent definitions of nursing knowledge suggest:

> *Nursing knowledge is the means by which the whole purpose of caring for patients is achieved because it underpins what we actually do.*
> (Hall, 2005, p34)
>
> *Nursing knowledge is drawn from a multifaceted base and includes evidence that comes from science (research and evaluation), experience and personally derived understanding.*
> (Moule and Goodman, 2009, p15)

From this perspective nursing knowledge stems from implementing both theory and practice, including psychosocial and cultural elements as well as practical processes. Patient assessment therefore also draws on the expertise of the nurse in being able to evaluate what is helpful, and what is less so, within the assessment process. Such reflective processes help to add to your knowledge base and develop your practice as a professional.

It is important for you to clarify the focus of the assessment in order for patients to be able to respond appropriately. This requires you to start from a position of understanding your own feelings about the assessment and the patient, as these can influence the assessment process and be revealed by your body language. The following case study offers an example of a nurse needing to control her own feelings when assessing the needs of a patient.

Case study: Toni's child assessment

Toni was in her first year of child nursing. She was working with her mentor Karen on a children's ward in an acute hospital. Toni had previously been shown how to carry out an initial admission assessment and so was completing the assessment under supervision today.

Emily was five years old and was being admitted from accident and emergency (A&E) with a broken leg following a fall. The A&E nurse told Karen and Toni privately that there was some suspicion that the fall might not have been accidental. Toni began the assessment by checking how Emily was feeling. However, Toni found it difficult to maintain eye contact with Emily's mother when she was asking her the assessment

> questions. Emily's mother responded by giving short answers. A few times Karen had to intervene to find out more information. Afterwards, Karen discussed with Toni how she thought the assessment had gone. Toni said she felt that she had got the relevant information, but found it difficult to talk to the mother because of thinking how Emily might have broken her leg. Karen explained how she had observed Toni's non-verbal communication betraying her judgement of Emily's mother, which affected her responses and the patient assessment. Karen emphasised the need to suppress our personal feelings in order to get the necessary information and to give unbiased care. Toni acknowledged that she found this a hard lesson to learn.

The case study above illustrates how personal feelings can sometimes cloud our judgement. Completing Activity 2.2 will help you to examine your own feelings about some of the different patients you might encounter.

Activity 2.2 — Reflection

Make a list of potential situations where you might find it difficult to provide unbiased care for a patient. Now reflect on why you would find it difficult to care for them. What does the code of conduct say a nurse must do in such circumstances (see the NMC web link at the end of the chapter)?

Which of the 6Cs is most relevant and absent in the case study above?

Although this activity is based on your own experience, there is a limited answer at the end of the chapter.

Your experiences, or those of people close to you, are likely to have influenced the list you have made. For example, you might have included those who perpetrate domestic violence or other abuses. Being aware of your reactions is an important first step to being able to deal with them. Having the 6Cs at the forefront of your thinking can help you to modify your reactions to respond positively. If you have a number of patients to care for, you will also need to prioritise whose assessment is the most important to do first (Sully and Dallas, 2005), and if you are unable to control your reactions then you might leave a potentially challenging patient until later inappropriately. Nurses do need to make judgements about care needs but should not make judgements about people, as these can be based on assumption and therefore skew the accuracy of the patient assessment. The nurse's role in patient assessment is to work with patients to identify their nursing needs and preferences and to gather information on behalf of other professionals involved in the patient's care.

Why is accurate patient assessment so important?

Accurate patient assessment is important in order to plan appropriate care that meets the patient's needs. To be able to carry out an accurate patient assessment you may also need to employ assessment tools, e.g. a wound assessment tool, or a pressure-scoring system. These help to integrate important subjective information with objective data to produce an accurate profile of the patient's needs. You can read more about how to use subjective and objective information in Chapter 3 and about assessment tools in Chapter 4. The following case study illustrates why accurate patient assessment is so important.

> ### Case study: Khalid's assessment
>
> *Khalid is 88 years old and has lost mobility recently. He is cared for by his daughter at home. After a recent fall he has lost confidence and wants to stay mainly in bed. As a result he has developed a pressure sore on his sacrum. The district nurse Katarina is looking after him. Katarina has some holiday booked in the next week and Khalid's daughter has noticed him becoming agitated.*
>
> *Katarina is keen to ensure that her colleagues who are going to look after Khalid maintain the same regimen as she knows he does not like change. She is therefore careful to document the pressure ulcer score and any contributing factors as well as the wound dressing used. To aid with assessment she also takes a photograph with Khalid's consent so that all the assessment data can be reviewed subjectively and objectively.*
>
> *Khalid does not respond well to Gabby, Katarina's replacement, often refusing to co-operate. She calls another nurse Fatima to help out. Fatima changes the pressure ulcer dressing after 3 days and notes that it appears to look better. She is basing this on visual inspection. She documents the improvement and tells Khalid who is pleased.*
>
> *When Katarina is back from her holiday the first thing Khalid tells her is of the improvement in his pressure sore. When she inspects it and compares it to the photo she took Katarina notes that it has in fact enlarged at one edge. She is left with the dilemma of what to say to Khalid without compromising her colleague.*

The case study highlights that it is important to be able to assess changes objectively and accurately in order to provide appropriate treatment and accurate information, as well as document the care-planning process. When Fatima assessed Khalid the assessment was incomplete because she had based it on her subjective opinion and not included more objective information, such as the photo of the wound. Therefore, while the wound may have appeared to be getting better, the information about this which she gave to Khalid was inaccurate. Any wound assessment needs to encompass wound bed condition as well as wound size and nutritional factors. What makes assessment good is making sure the information collected is complete. This may involve other professionals who may have a different view of the assessment required but whose input to the overall evaluation of the problem is important (Field and Smith, 2008). Completing Activity 2.3 will help you to identify what other professionals might be involved in Khalid's care and how this fits in to the overall assessment.

Understanding our role in patient assessment

Activity 2.3 — Critical thinking

When thinking about Khalid's case, who else do you think might be involved in his care and what would they be assessing in particular? Ask your mentor who the tissue viability nurse is in your placement area and ask that individual what assessment strategies he or she uses.

Which of the 6Cs is most relevant to Khalid's case and why?

An outline answer is given at the end of the chapter.

Completing this activity should not only help you to identify other relevant professionals involved in Khalid's care, but also demonstrate the importance of integrating their different perspectives before planning care. Field and Smith (2008, p21) state that:

> *The aim is to avoid duplication of information and records and to stop professionals giving conflicting advice.*

It is important for patients to experience a seamless service if they are to be confident that their needs are being properly assessed and communicated. In Khalid's case, this means using validated standardised approaches to wound assessment or treatment. Most healthcare organisations have developed specific tools which are incorporated into their patient assessment documentation. These are based on research informing guidelines and organisational policy. Wound assessment charts vary between organisations, but commonly consider the dimensions of the wound, the appearance of the wound bed and surrounding skin, any exudate or bleeding, level of pain and location of the wound to be entered on the human diagram (Dougherty and Lister, 2011). The case study highlights that professionals need to be honest about any gaps in their understanding and explain to patients why they are pursuing certain avenues of enquiry because our ways of knowing vary.

Four ways of working with facts

Healthcare practice is uncertain because we are dealing with unique individuals who do not always respond in the way that we expect. It is important for health practitioners to be able to deal with this uncertainty constructively in order for patients to be able to trust them to provide the most appropriate care. When we are working we usually access our knowledge to try to make decisions about what to do. Girard (2007) identifies four ways of knowing. How this relates to dealing with facts is set out in Table 2.1 using Johari window principles to consider areas that are known, others we are blind to, some we have not yet discovered and others we are unaware of (Luft and Ingham, 1955, cited in Hillson and Murray-Webster, 2007, p116).

Being able to identify the four areas of factual knowledge is an important step to understanding how you think and how you can tap into knowledge that you might not know you have. Read the following case study and then complete Activity 2.4 in order to find out what you currently know and don't know and, more importantly, what else you need to know to understand patients' needs and give effective care.

Facts you know you know	Facts you know you don't know
Available information which you can use, e.g. the name and age of the patient and the patient's problem	Gaps in the information, where you know you need to find out more, e.g. what medication the patient takes/whether the patient has any allergies
Facts you know but don't know that you know	**Facts you don't know you don't know**
Knowledge you have but are not aware of until it is needed, e.g. how to deal with a fire	Information you are not aware that you need and need to discover, e.g. what to do about a patient's non-compliance

Table 2.1: Four areas of factual knowledge

Case study: Mr Haughton's admission

Mr Haughton is a 60-year-old man with leukaemia. He is admitted to the ward with pyrexia of 38.6°C and nausea. He has a history of a previous laparoscopic cholecystectomy 2 months ago. Mr Haughton has blood taken and an abdominal X-ray is done. He is started on IV fluids and antibiotics. After 10 days in hospital Mr Haughton is able to return home.

Activity 2.4   Reflection

Review Mr Haughton's case and try to identify how your knowledge fits into the four areas illustrated in Table 2.1.

An outline answer is given at the end of the chapter.

Mr Haughton's case highlights that patients may have a number of concurrent problems, and this makes assessing and caring for them complex. While you may have knowledge about some of these, there are also areas that you need to discover more about. Understanding that there are always gaps in our knowledge and that we need to be aware of areas we are ignorant of is an important aspect of understanding yourself in the assessment process and what you need to do. You might identify that you lack knowledge about the patient's condition or what decision to make. You might want to include others such as your mentor or another professional in your thinking and decision-making processes. Standing's (2014) cognitive continuum might offer some ideas about how we think about making decisions in practice (see Chapter 10 for more information on making decisions within patient assessment).

Standing's cognitive continuum and relevance to nurses and patient assessment

Making decisions when assessing patients means understanding the evidence base for practice. There are a number of modes of practice according to Standing (2014, p8). These are:

- intuitive judgement – sensing patient concerns and changes;
- reflective judgement – moment-by-moment reviewing and revising of your practice;
- patient and peer-aided judgement – reaching consensus decisions with the patient and others;
- system-aided judgement – making use of policies and assessment tools;
- critical review of experience and research evidence – critical evaluation of your experience and available research that underpins this;
- action research and clinical audit – evaluating practice against benchmarks;
- qualitative research – interpreting the patient experience;
- survey research – making use of trends of evidence within particular populations;
- experimental research – identifying generalisable evidence.

It is important for you to know what evidence you are drawing upon within patient assessment and care planning in order to ensure that you can justify the decisions you make to the patient and to the profession. This will be discussed further in Chapter 10, but we begin here with a case study and an activity to help you critically consider your current knowledge and skills.

Case study: Lily's bowel problem

Lily is 45 years old and has recently been having problems with some urgency and faecal incontinence. She has seen her GP who has diagnosed irritable bowel disease and as part of her care refers Lily to the specialist bladder and bowel nurse. Lily is seen by Nicky, the specialist bladder and bowel nurse, who takes a full history and asks Lily to keep a diary of her diet and fluid intake and bladder and bowel action. She also completes a bladder scan, which is normal. Nicky asks Lily to look at the Bristol stool chart and identify which best matches her normal stool appearance. Lily identifies that her stools best match types 4 and 5, which are smooth and soft, sometimes too soft. Nicky advises Lily that she needs to cut down on her fruit intake and explains ways for Lily to manage her occasional faecal incontinence. Nicky makes an appointment to see Lily again in six weeks.

In the case study, Nicky, the specialist bladder and bowel nurse, has gathered her evidence through talking to Lily about her history and eating habits, identified precisely the type of stool Lily is producing and used her knowledge of research and practice to advise Lily on a plan of action. When completing an assessment, if we simply said to patients, 'You need to stop eating so much fruit', they would be understandably reluctant unless we can provide the evidence for our recommendation. Completing Activity 2.5 will help you to explore how you might use the different modes in your own practice.

> **Activity 2.5** — *Reflection*
>
> Think about your last placement and the different patients you nursed. Consider in what circumstances you can identify using a particular mode from Standing's (2014) continuum. Why was this mode of practice particularly relevant to the situation?
>
> *Although this activity is based on your own experience, there is a limited answer at the end of the chapter.*

You might have considered using an assessment tool to help gain further information, or reviewing how you were communicating with the patient. Less obvious is how we justify the thinking processes we employ, to come to the decisions we make. It is important to understand these thinking processes ourselves so we can explain them to the patient and to other health professionals, to justify the courses of action we propose. With this level of evidence patients might be more inclined and informed to consider their response. However, it is important to recognise the subjective nature of truth in terms of what patients tell us and what we think is important. Completing Activity 2.6 will help you to understand that the truth we are seeking in patient assessment is what patients' needs are and the most effective way to help them.

> **Activity 2.6** — *Reflection*
>
> Reflect on how a variety of evidence is used to help understand what help a patient may need and how best to provide it.
>
> *An outline answer is given at the end of the chapter.*

Part of patient decision-making is therefore also about evaluating the nature of what patients are telling us. The following case study will illustrate this point.

The nature of truth

> **Case study: Petia's pain experience**
>
> *Petia was a learning-disabled teenager living in a residential community setting. She complained of stomach cramps during her normal menstruation and was usually given paracetamol by the staff. Petia was admitted to the local hospital for a minor procedure. A carer came with her but could not stay*

> all the time. Petia became distressed when she was in pain. The staff on the ward tried to calm her, but Petia got more and more distressed. Petia was given pain medication but not as frequently as she could have it as the staff assumed that her agitation was part of her normal behaviour. The assessment tool they used was for children. Petia was left unnecessarily in pain because the staff did not believe her and had made assumptions about her.

What Petia's case study highlights is that we may use our own pain experience or behavioural norms to interpret that of others, rather than accepting the truth taken from their perspective. In doing so we may use stereotyping assumptions for interpretation. Equally, the case study illustrates some of the consequences when communication, care and competence – 3 of the 6Cs – have not been sufficiently applied.

Truth is determined by ourselves in accordance with our values and beliefs, by others and how influential we perceive them to be and by society. For example, those perceived to be in a powerful position, such as doctors, may not be questioned about their version of the truth. In mental health nursing we might call into question the singular nature of reality when many patients experience something very different. Therefore, truth remains tentative and uncertain and subjective in nature. Sometimes, when truth is perceived to be what is expressed by another, the subjective view is discounted, closing down the ability to look at personal experience (Frosh, 2002). What this means is that if professionals impose their interpretation of the patient's experience on to the patient, it is less likely that patients will be able to tell what their actual experience is and they may just go along with what the professional suggests. Decisions based on such a flawed perspective will then be compromised, including any care that is planned.

Stereotyping

Stereotyping is a way of categorising things and people which allows us to draw on previous experiences of those categories to direct our actions, which is quicker than forming new categories (Goodman and Clemow, 2010). However, the negative effect of stereotyping is making assumptions about another person which may not be accurate. We stereotype based on our personal values, beliefs and experiences, and this may relate to patients, colleagues and peers. For example, if we saw a man weaving along the street looking dishevelled, we might stereotype him as being drunk, even though there are many neurological reasons why someone might be moving in that way. As highlighted in the case study of Petia, stereotyping can equally cause us to make inaccurate assumptions about why someone is behaving in a particular way. If a health professional is working from such an assumption patient assessment will be affected. Completing Activity 2.7 will help you to examine situations where you may have been stereotyping people.

Activity 2.7 — Reflection

Think about a recent practice experience where you think you might have been stereotyping someone and consider the following questions:

1. How did you stereotype the person?
2. Why do you think you were stereotyping that person?
3. What was the result of your stereotyping that individual?

As this activity is based on your personal experience, there is no outline answer at the end of the chapter.

You might be stereotyping by using norms for situations such as how to behave in class or in the professional setting and expectations of particular roles (Goodman and Clemow, 2010). However, if stereotyping results in diminishing someone else's choices, the effects are not helpful. We need to consider our own values and responses and adjust our professional behaviour.

Conclusion

Good patient assessment is the goal for the nurse because in order to provide good care we need to learn a lot about our patients. We can only do this by accessing and applying the full range of relevant evidence at our disposal. Nevertheless, it is also recognised that nurses and patients are individuals who have their own values and ideas which need to be reconciled in order for accurate patient assessment and care planning to ensue. This may sometimes be difficult to do, but in the process we can learn a lot about ourselves and become better professionals.

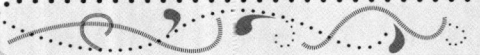

Chapter summary

This chapter has clarified what patient assessment is and highlighted some factors which are helpful and hindering to effective patient assessment, looking in particular at the influence of personal values and attitudes and application of the 6Cs. The activities included in the chapter have invited you to again consider your own values and beliefs because you need to grasp how influential these can be when you are assessing a patient. The chapter has also introduced Standing's (2014) nine modes of practice as a way of thinking about how you justify your thought processes and the decisions that you make. This will be discussed further in Chapter 10.

Activities: brief outline answers

Activity 2.1 Critical thinking [page 21]

Graham has not thought through the implications of Aaron's strict religious observance on food choices. A further dietician referral might be needed. Brett is accountable for this gap and by not following up the

Understanding our role in patient assessment

information could result in Aaron being at further risk of poor management of his diabetes when he leaves the hospital. Aaron's knowledge about how to manage his diabetes remains compromised due to his cultural needs not being adequately explored by Graham. This case study highlights how important commitment – one of the 6Cs – to the person is and not just the task being completed.

Activity 2.2 Reflection [page 23]

You might have included the following within your list:

- drunk driver;
- drug addict;
- paedophile;
- rapist;
- murderer;
- terrorist.

The NMC (2008, 2015) code of conduct is clear that all nurses must treat people as individuals. This means:

- you must treat people as individuals and respect their dignity;
- you must not discriminate in any way against those in your care;
- you must treat people kindly and considerately;
- you must act as an advocate for those in your care, helping them to access relevant health and social care, information and support.

Compassion – one of the 6Cs – is the most relevant here because it demonstrates drawing alongside someone and not judging them, but trying to discern their needs.

Activity 2.3 Critical thinking [page 25]

The other people involved in Khalid's's care are likely to be his GP, who will be overseeing the progress of his pressure ulcer. Khalid may also be assessed by a dietician who will be evaluating his nutritional needs and preferences. Khalid could also be assessed by the specialist tissue viability nurse, who will be monitoring the wound and healing specifically and offering advice on wound-dressing options. A multidisciplinary meeting would help to integrate these assessment processes but in the community setting comprehensive integrated notes are more often used for this purpose. Competence – one of the 6Cs – is the most relevant to this case in terms of how Fatima assessed Khalid's pressure ulcer.

Activity 2.4 Reflection [page 26]

The facts you know are Mr Haughton's age, the conditions he has come in with, his history of a laparoscopic cholecystectomy and that he is pyrexial. The facts you know you don't know are his normal medication, any allergies, what type of leukaemia he has and how it is normally treated and whether the pyrexia is due to his leukaemia or something going on with his previous surgery. The facts you don't know you know are about blood components and what they do and you can therefore link this to how Mr Haughton is likely to be affected by his leukaemia. The facts you don't know you don't know are likely to be related to Mr Haughton's healing response in the light of having leukaemia and any other aspects of his condition or care which you have not thought about.

Activity 2.5 Reflection [page 28]

You are likely to have used intuitive judgement such as realising that the patient is upset when you made your assessment and trying to understand the patient's response. At the same time you are likely to have reflected on your own communication – one of the 6Cs – with the patient and how perhaps your tone of voice allowed that person to open up to you. You will have needed to interpret the patient's experience from what he or she told you. You may have needed to consult with your mentor about the assessment or care-planning process as well as checking whether the patient was in agreement with what you planned. Using an assessment tool such as the Bristol stool chart might have helped you to collect accurate detail on which to base your clinical judgement. When evaluating your practice experience more broadly, such as for your portfolio, you may have considered how your practice fits with the NMC standards and the 6Cs and what you are actually using to underpin what you do. You may have read up on cancer treatments and how successful these are for certain types of cancer.

Chapter 2

Activity 2.6 Reflection [page 28]

You might have included:

- the story/history that the patient gives about a need or problem;
- nursing observations;
- assessment tool results;
- peer-aided judgements such as discussion with your mentor, or multidisciplinary meeting outcomes;
- research findings;
- policies and guidelines.

Further reading

Goodman, B and Clemow, R (2010) *Nursing and Collaborative Practice: A Guide to Interprofessional Learning and Working*, 2nd edn. Exeter: Learning Matters.

A useful book for understanding how professionals' values can influence their approach to patients and each other and guidance on how to work more collaboratively.

Standing, M (2014) *Clinical Judgement and Decision-Making for Nursing Students*, 2nd edn. London: SAGE Publications.

This book introduces decision-making theory and its relevance to nursing practice.

Useful website

www.nmc-uk.org

The website of the Nursing and Midwifery Council – where you can find a great deal of professional information including the latest guidance on the code of conduct for nurses and midwives.

Chapter 3
Making sense of patient information

Lioba Howatson-Jones

NMC Standards for Pre-registration Nursing Education

This chapter will address the following competencies:

Domain 2: Communication and interpersonal skills
3. All nurses must use the full range of communication methods, including verbal, non-verbal and written, to acquire, interpret and record their knowledge and understanding of people's needs. They must be aware of their own values and beliefs and the impact this may have on their communication with others. They must take account of the many different ways in which people communicate and how these may be influenced by ill health, disability and other factors, and be able to recognise and respond effectively when a person finds it hard to communicate.

Domain 3: Nursing practice and decision-making
7. All nurses must be able to recognise and interpret signs of normal and deteriorating mental and physical health and respond promptly to maintain or improve the health and comfort of the service user, acting to keep them and others safe.

NMC Essential Skills Clusters (ESCs)

This chapter will address the following ESCs:

Cluster: Care, compassion and communication
6. People can trust the newly registered graduate nurse to engage therapeutically and actively listen to their needs and concerns, responding by using skills that are helpful, providing information that is clear, accurate, meaningful and free from jargon.

By the first progression point:
1. Communicates effectively both orally and in writing, so that the meaning is always clear.
2. Records information accurately and clearly on the basis of observation and communication.
3. Effectively communicates people's stated needs and wishes to other professionals.

By the second progression point:
4. Uses strategies to enhance communication and remove barriers to effective communication, minimising risk to people from lack of or poor communication

Chapter 3

> **Chapter aims**
>
> After reading this chapter you should be able to:
>
> - differentiate between the nurse's and other health professionals' roles in gathering patient information;
> - identify when gathering information could be difficult;
> - differentiate between different types and forms of information;
> - identify different questioning techniques;
> - analyse a variety of patient information in order to identify nursing priorities for action;
> - make sense of the information received from patients through checking accuracy of understanding, and be able to interpret and explain this to others.

Introduction

> **Case study: Mr White's recent hospital visit**
>
> *James White is 55 years old and has had a number of investigations and short admissions over the past few years. He is brought to your placement ward with epigastric pain (pain in the upper abdominal region). He has quite a thick file of notes. He has had blood taken, an electrocardiogram (ECG), which is a tracing of the electrical activity of the heart, and baseline nursing observations. Your mentor suggests that you talk to Mr White to find out how he is feeling and what he understands as being the problem. In the meantime your mentor asks you to repeat the nursing observations, checks through the notes for his history and the computer for his blood result. Mr White tells you that he has previously had an oesophageal gastroduodenoscopy (OGD), a procedure where a telescopic camera is passed down the food pipe and through the stomach into the small intestine. This investigation found a small ulcer which he thinks might be what is causing him pain. He also tells you that he recently lost his job and has been drinking a bit more than usual because he feels so low. Your mentor tells you that his blood count indicates that he is anaemic, which means his blood cells have less oxygen-carrying capacity. His ECG is normal. When you complete his nursing observations you note that his pulse is a bit raised, which could also mean he is bleeding from somewhere. Subsequently Mr White has a further OGD which indicates that the ulcer has enlarged and has been bleeding. Following a blood transfusion his medication is increased and he is advised to cut down his alcohol intake and is discharged home.*

No matter how long or short their history, a great variety of information is gathered from patients when they enter the health and social care setting. As the above case study identifies, this information needs to be interpreted swiftly and accurately. It is part of the nurse's role to make sense of this information by checking with the patient and others and to use it accurately in order to plan appropriate care with the patient. In the above case study the nurse checks with Mr White what his view of the problem is and the accuracy of the history that can be found in the notes and integrates this with nursing observations and test results. As a student you need to be able to gather relevant patient information and interpret it by identifying its meaning and significance and referring to other health professionals. This is important for developing your communication competence with others.

This chapter will start by defining patient information, identifying the roles of different healthcare professionals in gathering patient information, and categorising different forms of information identifying the strengths and weaknesses of these categories. The chapter will consider the appropriateness of different questioning techniques such as open, closed, probing and laddering questions. A variety of activities are offered to encourage you to make sense of information, identify situations that make gathering information difficult, differentiate the role of the nurse from that of other healthcare professionals, and learn how to analyse information in order to act on it. Through these activities you will be asked to reflect on the assessment process.

What is patient information?

Patient information can be defined as any information that relates to a patient. This will include personal details as well as those relating to health status and social context. It is gathered by health professionals for the purpose of helping the patient in some way. Different fields of practice broadly focus on different aspects of information. For example, mental health is very concerned with psychosocial elements. Therefore information relating to family history, behaviour, mood, mental state, recreational activities and relationships is all deemed particularly relevant and important. Occupational therapy is concerned with what individuals can do for themselves while physiotherapists focus upon information relating to mobility and issues that affect it. Both professional groups are interested in rehabilitating the patient. Therefore patient capabilities and preferences are the main focus. Social work considers the social context, particularly in relation to vulnerability. Medicine is concerned with identifying the medical problem and finding solutions. This can be described as taking a deficit view, although many doctors do now take part in health promotion activities as well. Because of nurses' unique position of close and regular contact with patients, they are able to co-ordinate making sense of information with patients, interpreting terms and explaining aspects they do not understand. This offers the opportunity for achieving a more holistic perspective which takes account of the patient's views as well as integrating a variety of professional opinion, as appropriate. 'Holistic' means a complete view which involves the patient. We proceed now to consider different types and forms of patient information. See Howatson-Jones and Ellis (2008) for further reading on what information is gathered where.

Different types and forms of information

Information can be divided into subjective and objective information. This can also be related to intuitive forms of thinking versus more rational and analytical forms of assessment (Standing, 2014). For example, in the case study about Mr White, objective information has been obtained from the nursing observations, the ECG and the blood results, which give a physiological view of the problem. Equally important, however, is the subjective information which Mr White has conveyed about how he is feeling and what he perceives the problem to be. Through this line of questioning other important information about his low mood and increased drinking is discovered. The importance of using both types of information in order to interpret accurately what is really happening with the patient is illustrated.

Subjective information relates to the descriptions that patients give of their experience and understanding of the situation. Your interpretation skills add another form of subjective information based on your professional experience. For example, when a patient describes a pain experience you will be observing that patient's non-verbal behaviour as well as listening to the description. It is likely that you will also be filtering your interpretation of the patient's pain experience through your intuitive knowledge of what is going on.

The weakness of relying solely on subjective information is that it is based on particular experience and may miss other important cues of what is going on. Objective information is quantitative data which can be measured; for example, vital signs such as pulse and blood pressure and tests such as blood results, which list the levels of different blood cells and blood constituents. The weakness of relying solely on objective information is that it signals an alteration has taken place, but does not identify how this affects the person. The main types of information gathered from patients and potential sources are given in Table 3.1, although this list is not exhaustive.

Subjective and objective information may also appear in different forms:

- Repeated information – this often comes from family and friends or carers who reinforce and help to elaborate the patient's story. For example, what tests the patient has had and what they have been told.
- Observation – this information is gathered by closely observing the patient, for example, being aware of the quality of the patient's breathing, how the patient is moving, and the patient's mood.
- Clinical information – this emerges from clinical activity with the patient, for example, recording observations, doing a wound dressing, and checking pressure areas.

A good patient assessment involves gathering a mix of both forms of information and using your senses – your eyes to observe patient behaviours, movement and how the patient looks, your ears to listen to breathing and what the patient is really saying, touch to feel what is revealed by the skin and smell to detect odours (Howatson-Jones, 2008). This information remains subjective and is also reliant on nursing experience. Therefore, it is also important to integrate objective information in order to underpin subjective interpretation. For this reason, when checking someone's pressure areas you will use your visual observation as well as the Waterlow screening tool in order to assess for risk factors you cannot see. The following two case studies illustrate what can happen if health professionals do not integrate the subjective with the objective but focus on one aspect only. Inexperience can result in unrealistic solutions.

Subjective	Part subjective, part objective	Objective
Biographical details – usually sourced from patients themselves but if they are incapacitated in some way, information may be obtained from family/friends/carers or from documentary evidence	Medical history – a chronological sequence of events taken by a doctor and which integrates relevant test results with physical examination. Usually uses a biomedical focus on the problem (see **www.gpnotebook.co.uk** or **www.evidence.nhs.uk** for the type of information sought)	Test results – sourced from diagnostic and interventional techniques which examine anatomical and physiological activity within narrow margins of normal and abnormal. These have usually developed from clinical trials – the highest level of research evidence (Ellis, 2013). Test modalities and retrieval involve technology requiring healthcare professionals to be health informatics-literate to access and process results (Hutchfield, 2010)
Social context – usually sourced from patient but often added to by family/friends/carers and by healthcare professional assessment such as occupational therapist, social worker community nursing and care managers	Referral information – sourced from a variety of healthcare professionals, including general practitioners, specialist doctors/nurses, occupational therapists, physiotherapists, mental health teams, social workers, care managers, speech therapists and dieticians and will also include any relevant test and observation results	
Symptoms – sourced from the patient but may be added to by family/friends/carers (**www.patients.uptodate.com**)	Prescription – sourced from general practitioner/patient/family/carer. Pharmacist will review before dispensing	
Observations – sourced from a variety of healthcare professionals, including nurses, occupational therapists, physiotherapists, dieticians, doctors and others		

Table 3.1: Types of information and potential sources

> ### Case study: Mrs Wu's diabetic control
>
> *Mrs Wu has type 2 diabetes, which is a long-term condition for which she takes tablets. She mostly manages this herself at home but her general practitioner has called her for a regular review at the surgery. A blood test is taken for glycohaemoglobin. This is a test which measures the amount of glucose bound to haemoglobin and can be an accurate measure of the average levels of blood glucose in the preceding three months and therefore the level of glucose control. The result came back as 10.3%, which is significantly raised. The normal levels are between 2.5 and 6.0%, and with moderate diabetic control 6.1–8.0% (Evans et al., 2003). Mrs Wu's medication was reviewed and she was referred to a dietician for further dietary advice. No one was aware that during this time Mrs Wu's husband had left her. The stress of this is likely to have contributed to the raised blood glucose levels through the release of glucocorticoids, which are hormones released by stress. While the interventions chosen might be relevant, they do not address the main problem, which is Mrs Wu's stress level.*

> ### Case study: Angelina's adaptation needs
>
> *Angelina is in her 70s and lives alone at home. She has been having difficulty getting about and washing and is generally finding it harder to manage. She is visited by an occupational therapist who is relatively new. Angelina tells the occupational therapist what she would like. The occupational therapist completes her patient assessment and identifies that Angelina requires a number of aids and alterations to help her continue to live a relatively independent life. Her recommendations are for grab hand rails to be fitted and the bathroom to be converted into a wet room shower and for a stairlift to be installed. Angelina is delighted with these proposals. However Angelina is less happy when the occupational therapist returns the following week to say that perhaps they need to start by trying out some hand rails on the stairs first and look at other ways of helping Angelina with washing. The occupational therapist's lack of experience had meant that her subjective view of the situation was unrealistic and that she set up expectations which could not be met.*

As demonstrated in the two case studies, focusing on the subjective and objective separately means that important patient information is missed and is not considered in planning interventions. They also demonstrate the importance of working with patients and their carers (if relevant) and not planning care from a purely professional viewpoint. We proceed now to consider when patients should be assessed.

When to assess patients

Patients need to be assessed at key points in their care journey. It is important to assess patients when they first identify they have a need, when meeting them for the first time, when their needs change, and when accepting, referring or discharging them. Where different healthcare practitioners are involved it may also be necessary to complete different assessments, although increasingly healthcare teams are becoming integrated. This is particularly true of the interface between acute and community care where the purpose of integrated teams is to reduce the assessment burden on the patient and promote a seamless service. Therefore it may be possible that a therapist or a nurse undertakes some of the patient assessments. Situations which can make patient assessment difficult are those where the patient is not capable of responding or where patient response is impaired in some way. Completing the following activity will help you to think about some situations where this could be the case.

> **Activity 3.1** *Critical thinking*
>
> Make a list of situations in which you think it is important for patients to be assessed.
>
> What situations might make gathering information from the patient difficult and what other methods might you use instead?
>
> *An outline answer is given at the end of the chapter.*

We proceed now to consider some questioning techniques when gathering patient information.

Questioning techniques

A good questioning technique is important to enable the patient to understand what is being asked and for the health professional to gain the information required to inform diagnostic and therapeutic processes. It is imperative to build a good therapeutic relationship and trust before launching into questioning. Egan (2014) identifies that important communication skills such as attentive listening, being open, responding and reflecting are needed to help people tell their story and to develop dialogue that gets to the core of the matter through probing and which aids understanding through summarising (Bach and Grant, 2011). The way you respond to a patient the first time you meet that person sets the tone for the rest of the encounter and therefore is crucial to establishing trust and dialogue. Take some time to complete Activity 3.2 and reflect on your communication with new patients. Also see McCabe and Timmins (2013) for further reading around communication techniques.

> **Activity 3.2** *Reflection*
>
> Reflect on previous encounters you have had with new patients and consider the following questions:
>
> 1. What went well and what did not go so well?
> 2. Why might this have been?
> 3. What strategies might you use going forward?
> 4. How can you help patients who have difficulty in supplying information?
>
> *As this activity is based on your experience, there is no outline answer given at the end of the chapter.*

Chapter 3

Reflecting on your own patient encounters may have highlighted that it is not always easy to elicit information and relying on your current communication skills may not be enough. If you have not had much experience in practice, the following case study may help you to consider some of the issues involved in communicating with patients.

> **Case study: Johann's questioning experience**
>
> *Johann was on a learning disability placement in his first year of his nurse preparation programme. He had no experience of communicating with someone with a learning disability. He was always fearful of triggering an outburst as he had heard from his peers of that happening sometimes.*
>
> *Johann tried to think of things to say, but found that people seemed to avoid him. When reflecting on this with his mentor Jenny, Johann identified that his non-verbal approaches were probably conveying his fear and making people avoid engaging with him. Johann and Jenny considered some strategies to overcome this.*
>
> - What strategies might you employ in a similar situation? Which of the 6Cs might this case study relate to?
>
> *There is an outline answer at the end of the chapter.*

As this case study demonstrates, it is helpful to learn the art of asking questions. Nolan and Ellis (2008) describe a number of questioning techniques that nurses can employ. These include open questions, where patients are able to choose how to frame their answer; closed questions, where the answer is limited; and probing questions, which seek more specific information. Best avoided are multiple questions, which are often used to query related problems. For example, asking about the nature of a particular symptom and what causes and relieves it in one sentence is likely to leave the patient confused. Similarly, leading questions which already contain the answer will elicit that answer from the patient as well as suppressing the patient's experience and will therefore not provide anything new. It needs to be remembered that when patients are in an unfamiliar setting they may not be able to respond as quickly or as thoughtfully as usual and will often rely on the nurse's skills to help them relay the necessary information. Probing questions are useful for focusing on specific issues or expanding answers. Rhetorical questions are statements which do not require an answer and may be used as ice breakers. For example, commenting on the weather may be useful to start to relax the patient and build a dialogue. However, such statements also need to be used with caution in order not to make people feel they are being patronised. Other more useful ice breakers could be used, such as introducing yourself and checking whether the patient has any questions.

Different categories of question are useful for different stages of the assessment process because they serve different functions. Table 3.2 offers some examples.

Questioning may also identify areas that are outside your current scope of knowledge and require you to refer to others. Activity 3.3 will help you to identify the interplay of different forms of questioning.

Making sense of patient information

Stage of nursing process	Type of question	Question content
Establishing baseline information	Closed questions	Can elicit biographical information such as name, date of birth, address, occupation, doctor, next of kin, whether a symptom is present or not, whether a procedure is consented to or not
Problem identification	Open questions	Useful for gaining understanding of the reason for requiring health and social care intervention, symptomatic description, personal management of the problem
Defining the problem	Probing questions	Can elicit what causes or alleviates the problem, clarification of patient explanation

Table 3.2: Types of questioning used in the nursing process

Activity 3.3 — Communication

Read the transcript below and identify where different forms of questions are being used.

Student: Good morning, Mrs Riley. My name is Emma and I am a student nurse. Welcome to the ward. I have a few questions that I need to ask you about your personal details and why you have come here today. Would that be all right?

Patient: Yes.

Student: Let's start with your details. What is your full name? Patient: My full name is Patricia Anne Riley.

Student: And do you like to be called Patricia, Anne or Mrs Riley or something shorter?

Patient: I prefer to be called Patricia.

Student: What is your address?

Patient: I live at 27 Long View Road, Brigstown, East Sussex.

Student: What is your telephone number?

Patient: 01443 56789.

Student: Who is your next of kin?

Patient: John Riley, my husband.

Student: Does he live at the same address and have the same telephone number?

Patient: He has a mobile number, which is 07798 45607.

Student: What has brought you here today?

Chapter 3

continued ...

> Patient: I have been having these terrible pains when I go to the toilet and I have been passing rather a lot of blood recently.
>
> Student: When you say going to the toilet, do you mean passing urine or having your bowels open?
>
> Patient: I mean having my bowels open.
>
> Student: Is there anything that you have noticed that makes the pain worse?
>
> Patient: When I eat spicy foods.
>
> Student: I presume you pass blood then as well? Have you been told what the problem might be?
>
> Patient: The doctor said something about irritable bowel syndrome but also having to rule out other causes and needing to do some more tests.
>
> Student: Did you understand what the doctor said?
>
> Patient: Not really.
>
> Student: Would you like me to get my mentor to help explain what irritable bowel syndrome is and the tests that the doctor has ordered?
>
> Patient: Yes please.
>
> *An outline answer is given at the end of the chapter.*

Price (2002) suggests that questions should be 'laddered', by which he means that they start from the least invasive questions about actions to the more invasive ones about beliefs and values. Laddering questions enables others to follow your focus and you to gain more in-depth information during a patient interview. Making use of reflective prompt cues can also be helpful. For example:

- Why – 'Why were you seeing your GP?'
- What – 'What were you doing just before the pain started?'
- Where – 'Where did you feel the burning sensation?'
- When – 'When do you feel the pain sensation?'
- Who – 'Who helps you with your care?'

Completing Activity 3.4 will help you to practise different questioning techniques in a safe environment as well as consider your style of communication.

Activity 3.4 — *Communication*

> This activity is designed to enable you to practise different questioning techniques in order to gain an understanding of why and how information might be withheld by people and explore what you might do about this.

Making sense of patient information

> 1. Spend about 15 minutes finding out as much as possible about the health of a peer or a family member.
> 2. Now compare the questions you asked with those you might ask as a health professional.
> 3. Were there any differences and why might this be?
> 4. What further information do you need?
> 5. Did you suspect that some information was being withheld?
> 6. What alerted you to this and what did you do?
>
> *An outline answer is given at the end of the chapter.*

Gathering information can be problematic for a number of reasons. Some of these are listed below.

- Knowing what you are looking for and understanding what it means – this is likely to be related to the reason why you are seeing the patient in the first place, but will also be related to professional experience. Those who are less experienced may not know how to assess for particular problems.
- Accurate recording and documentation – if records are not kept accurately and recorded in a timely manner, important information may be missing.
- Patient memory and ability to articulate it – patients may not be able to remember key points or be able to explain them. This is where asking a carer or family member can help to get a picture of the problem.
- Technology – technological breakdown can mean that important information is not accessible.
- Institutional differences – ways of collecting, collating and storing information can vary between institutions, making it difficult to make sense of some of the information that healthcare professionals have gathered.
- Archiving – archives can sometimes be difficult to access.

Patients may also not always be truthful in the information they give because of their own agendas. For example, ambulatory care settings, where people require care for less than 24 hours, often require there to be a responsible adult at home with the patient following certain procedures or day surgery. A patient may not want to admit that there is no one because he or she wants to go home. Equally, the patient may be afraid that the procedure will not go ahead. And yet if something goes wrong at home as a consequence, the communication, assessment and decision-making processes of the nurse will also be scrutinised. It is therefore important to reflect on your own problem-solving and identify what options are available to you. Identifying nursing priorities is the next step after talking to the patient. We move forward now to consider areas to focus upon when analysing patient information.

Identifying nursing priorities through analysis of patient information

Part of the nurse's role is to analyse the information received from the patient, and by other means, such as from carers and patient notes, in order to identify what needs to be done.

Carpenito-Moyet (2010, p52) suggests three main areas of focus when analysing patient information for nursing priorities:

1. strengths – areas which the patient can draw upon to progress to a previous or new health state;
2. risk factors – those things which might hold the patient back from recovery or progression;
3. problems in functioning – areas which are not working properly.

A case study is offered to illustrate these points.

Scenario: Ella's loss of sense of self

Ella Livesey is 45 and has come in to the neurological unit because of a multiple sclerosis (MS) relapse which has affected her mobility, sight and bladder and bowel control. She has had MS for 15 years and is usually relatively self-caring between relapses. She has had six relapses in the last 15 years. The last two relapses have had a profound effect on her mobility each time, which is why she has been admitted to hospital. She is also due to receive a course of intravenous medication to try to deal with some of the effects of the relapse.

You are the nurse admitting Ella. You observe that she is using two sticks to walk, is very wobbly and uncoordinated and appears to be taking time to absorb information and answer your questions. When you ask her to remove her cardigan so that you can record her blood pressure she fumbles with the buttons. You start to think:

- *What are the significant nursing features?*
- *What is the patient's nursing care priority?*

You identify that Ella has had MS for 15 years and therefore has built up her knowledge and coping strategies for dealing with the illness (strengths to draw on). You start by asking her what her immediate concerns are. She identifies that, although her mobility has been badly affected, of greater concern to her is her loss of bladder and bowel control, which has altered her view of herself as a woman and a wife (problems with functioning). She feels that without that sense of identity she cannot deal with her other losses, i.e. mobility and visual acuity. Previously she has always been able to problem-solve and look forward with hope to recovery and a return to a degree of normality. This time she is not so sure and feels hopeless (risk factors).

Together you identify that the first priority is to involve the continence nurse to seek options and solutions. You discuss how she might cultivate a positive outlook to aid her recovery. You also consider how to solve functional problems by identifying what help she desires with washing and dressing and where to place the furniture to avoid obstacles and how she might involve her husband in helping. You suggest the input of the occupational therapist for further advice on how to maintain her independent living. Finally you discuss the planned medical treatment and its potential side effects and what she might want to do to aid her recovery further when she goes home.

How might the 6Cs relate to this scenario?

There is an outline answer at the end of the chapter.

The aspects relating to coping mechanisms, functional problems and altered self-image, as demonstrated in the case study, can then form the basis of your analysis of nursing priorities. Completing Activity 3.5 will help you think about the nursing priorities in relation to Ella's case study.

> **Activity 3.5** *Communication*
>
> Read the scenario above about Ella again. How would you configure the nursing priorities within the scenario for a nursing handover?
>
> *There is an outline answer at the end of the chapter.*

Not all aspects will fall within your scope of practice or expertise and therefore will require onward referral or notification to other health and social care professionals such as the doctor or occupational therapist. It is important that nurses are able to reach agreement with the patient about what these priorities are as part of patient-centred care which does not treat patients as objects, but as people concerned with their health and wellbeing and as collaborators in care. Working in such a way has been described as a skilled relationship which is based on viewing people as being in relationship with themselves, with those around them, the situation and the larger world (Dewing, 2004; McCormack, 2004).

As the case study demonstrates, working with the patient is important, but also something that can become lost in the busy healthcare environment. And yet, how can we expect patients to self-manage if they are not involved in their care decision-making? As the healthcare environment changes and more patients are cared for in the community in their own homes, supporting them in their self-management is increasingly important. Consequently nursing priorities need to reflect and incorporate patient priorities in order to promote the continuity of care and recovery. Having identified nursing priorities, it is important to be able to explain these accurately to the patient and to be able to make sense of this explanation to other health professionals interpreting any specialist terms. The following section considers how to make sense of patient information.

Making sense of information and interpreting this to others

Professionals need to focus on becoming what Egan (2014, p29) calls 'translator-practitioners'. What this means is having a good understanding of the relevant research and evidence base as well as the practical possibilities in order to be able to communicate accurately with patients and other health professionals and to make sense of this for both professionals and patients in terms that are understandable to them. Interpretation here means being able to interpret terms that may be profession-specific as well as give an explanation of how they apply. Questions that you might want to ask yourself as part of this process are:

- What is the patient's reason for admission, or the patient's explanation/understanding for his or her current situation?
- What are the trends and significance within the objective information available?
- What is the important subjective information in this case and what does it tell you?
- Is there further information that you need?
- How do you develop a handover report?

Reading the case study below and then completing Activity 3.6 will help you to identify the key points which need to be considered and passed on within a given situation.

Case study: Robert's deteriorating health

Robert is a 65-year-old man who has chronic kidney disease and related hypertension. His condition has slowly been deteriorating and he has recently become quite depressed. He has difficulty sleeping and feels quite weak. He is under the care of the specialist community matron team where you are currently on placement.

He tells you that his wife normally takes care of him but due to financial pressures she has had to take a part-time job. He feels deprived of company. His blood pressure readings are significantly raised and when you check the nursing notes you see that these have been steadily rising. You note that he has had a recent blood test but does not know the result. He has an appointment in the dialysis clinic scheduled for next week.

Activity 3.6 — Critical thinking

List the important points you have identified from your interactions with Robert.

How would you formulate a documentary entry for informing other professionals about his situation and progress?

An outline answer is given at the end of the chapter.

Making sense of information means making sure you understand it all in the first place. For example, do you know what causes chronic kidney disease and the effects it can have on people? Have you checked with Robert what he understands and how he copes? Do you know the management processes involved? Unless you understand the results of your questions you cannot explain these to the patient and to other health professionals like the clinic nurse who Robert is going to see. Having made sense of a patient's information it is also important to identify the nursing priorities in order to start formulating a care plan.

Conclusion and reflection

Finding all the patient information needed can sometimes be a process of detection as you follow up different cues and leads. This involves communicating not only with the patient, but also with a variety of people, often across different disciplines.

Reflection will enable you to develop your practice by tracking changes in the way you think and act and make sense of your responses (Howatson-Jones, 2013). Completing Activity 3.7 will help you to make sense of how you gather and interpret information.

> **Activity 3.7**   *Reflection*
>
> Consider a recent experience where you were involved in gathering and interpreting patient information and answer the following questions.
>
> - How did you go about gathering and interpreting the information and what problems did you encounter?
> - How did you address any problems?
> - What other ways could you have used?
> - Would you do the same again and why?
>
> Having reflected on how you gather and interpret information, draw up an action plan of what you are taking forward. (You might like to refer to Howatson-Jones (2013), for further guidance on making use of reflection.)
>
> *As this activity is based on your own experiences, there is a limited outline answer at the end of the chapter.*

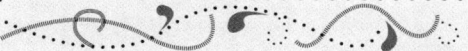

> **Chapter summary**
>
> The processes of gathering and interpreting information are important to ensure the accuracy of patient assessment and care planning. This chapter has highlighted some of the techniques involved in developing a process of questioning and of working with subjective and objective information. It has focused on how to interpret information to others involved in the patient's care and how to identify nursing priorities through analysis of the information received. You have been offered the opportunity to complete a variety of activities in order to help you to develop your communication and critical thinking skills and to reflect on how and why you carry out patient assessment and alternatives that might work differently.

> **Case studies: brief outline answers**
>
> **Johann's questioning experience [page 40]**
>
> *Some strategies which you might think about could be to approach people as persons and develop a conversation by finding out what their interests are and talking about those. Being yourself is important. You could talk about a few of your interests as well, if it seems appropriate. This case study relates to communication – one of the 6Cs.*

Chapter 3

continued ...

Ella's loss of sense of self [page 44]

This case study relates to a number of the 6Cs. These include commitment to Ella by finding out what her priorities are. Also, compassion through understanding her struggle; caring through identifying ways to help her with activities of daily living; competence in how the assessment is completed.

Activities: brief outline answers

Activity 3.1 Critical thinking [page 39]

Ideally, patients should be assessed continually. However there are some key points when assessment is recommended, such as at admission, pre- and post-procedures, when transferred and prior to discharge. Patient circumstances which might make this difficult are reduced mental capacity, level of consciousness, effects of drugs, language ability, effects of illness and trust. Other methods for gathering information which you might use are making use of your senses, intuition and medical devices such as monitors. You might also expand your sources to include family, friends and carers, as appropriate.

Activity 3.3 Communication [page 41]

Student:	Good morning, Mrs Riley. My name is Emma and I am a student nurse. Welcome to the ward. I have a few questions that I need to ask you about your personal details and why you have come here today. **Would that be all right? (closed question)**
Patient:	Yes.
Student:	Let's start with your details. **What is your full name? (closed question)**
Patient:	My full name is Patricia Anne Riley.
Student:	**And do you like to be called Patricia, Anne or Mrs Riley or something shorter? (closed question)**
Patient:	I am happy to be called Patricia.
Student:	**What is your address? (closed question)**
Patient:	I live at 27 Long View Road, Brigstown, East Sussex.
Student:	**What is your telephone number? (closed question)**
Patient:	01443 56789.
Student:	**Who is your next of kin? (closed question)**
Patient:	John Riley, my husband.
Student:	**Does he live at the same address and have the same telephone number? (multiple questions)**
Patient:	He has a mobile number, which is 07798 45607.
Student:	**What has brought you here today? (open question)**
Patient:	I have been having these terrible pains when I go to the toilet and I have been passing rather a lot of blood recently.
Student:	**When you say going to the toilet, do you mean passing urine or having your bowels open? (probing question)**

Patient:	I mean having my bowels open.
Student:	**Is there anything that you have noticed that makes the pain worse? (probing question)**
Patient:	When I eat spicy foods.
Student:	**I presume you pass blood then as well? (leading question) Have you been told what the problem might be? (closed question)**
Patient:	The doctor said something about irritable bowel syndrome but also having to rule out other causes and needing to do some more tests.
Student:	**Did you understand what the doctor said? (closed question)**
Patient:	Not really.
Student:	**Would you like me to get my mentor to help explain what irritable bowel syndrome is and the tests that the doctor has ordered? (closed question)**
Patient:	Yes please.

Activity 3.4 Communication [page 42]

You are likely to have used a more conversational and less formal questioning style with a peer or family member because your relationship is already established. Health professionals use more formal questioning techniques. You are likely to have been alerted to the withholding of information by a change in non-verbal behaviour, such as breaking of eye contact, fidgeting and breaks in sentence structure. Reasons for withholding information might be lack of trust, anxiety and not understanding the question. You might have thought of using reassurance, being open and honest about why you needed the information and what it would be used for and adjusting your position to one that was open.

Activity 3.5 Communication [page 45]

Ella Livesey is 45 years old and was admitted with an MS relapse. Some of the symptoms such as loss of mobility and loss of bladder control have been distressing for her. She has also been psychologically impacted by this abrupt change to her body image. I have assessed the nursing priorities to be helping Ella with maintaining a safe environment and to support her psychological adjustment to this new reality.

Activity 3.6 Critical thinking [page 46]

Robert is feeling depressed. The reasons might include a loss of self-esteem because his wife has to go to work in order to ease the financial burden. He appears to be missing her company. His blood pressure rise may be linked to these factors making him feel more stressed, but you also need to find out what the blood test was for and the result. Your documentary entry could go something like this:

> 01.04.2012: Attended Mr Watson today. His blood pressure was raised at 228/125 mmHg. The trend for this has been steadily rising over the last two weeks. He appeared lethargic and in a low mood today. On talking to him he seems to be missing his wife's company and feels isolated. He had blood taken on 29.03.12: Results are being sought. He has an appointment in the dialysis clinic on 08.04.2012. He may need a medication review and referral to the counsellor.

Activity 3.7 Reflection [page 47]

Action planning involves identifying what you have learned and relating this to what you intend to do in practice:

> Action plan: I had problems gathering patient information because the patient did not understand the terminology I was using. I changed my approach by using simpler terms but this meant that I needed to understand what I was saying and I was not clear on some areas myself. Next time I will make sure that I understand what I am trying to explain *before* I meet with patients. I intend to keep reading about this particular topic area and discuss with my mentor to ensure the accuracy of my understanding.

Further reading

Bach, S and Grant, A (2015) *Communication and Interpersonal Skills for Nurses*, 3rd edn. London: SAGE Publications.
A useful introduction to communication and interpersonal skills for nursing students.

Ellis, P (2013) *Evidence-Based Practice in Nursing*, 2nd edn. London: SAGE Publications.
This book clarifies what is meant by evidence-based practice and how you can find and apply it.

Howatson-Jones, L (2013) *Reflective Practice in Nursing*, 2nd edn. London: SAGE Publications.
A guide to the variety of ways in which you can reflect on your practice in order to develop and improve future practice.

Howatson-Jones, L and Ellis, P (eds) (2008) *Outpatient, Day Surgery and Ambulatory Care*. Chichester: Wiley-Blackwell.
This book outlines the nursing role and procedures in a variety of ambulatory and outpatient settings and will help to develop your knowledge of nursing contexts.

Hutchfield, K (2010) *Information Skills for Nursing Students*. Exeter: Learning Matters.
A clear description of where to source information and ways of doing this; this book will help you to be effective in your search for relevant information.

McCabe, C and Timmins, F (2013) *Communication Skills for Nursing Practice*, 2nd edn. Basingstoke: Palgrave Macmillan.
This book outlines the variety of ways in which nurses and midwives communicate with patients, each other and the wider team. It offers suggestions for developing your communication skills.

Useful websites

www.evidence.nhs.uk
This website links to the latest research and evidence about treatment for a variety of medical conditions.

www.gpnotebook.co.uk
This website is a reference source which patients and professionals can use.

www.patients.uptodate.com
This website offers information about various medical conditions.

Chapter 4
Assessment tools

Lioba Howatson-Jones

NMC Standards for Pre-registration Nursing Education

This chapter will address the following competencies:

Domain 3: Nursing practice and decision-making

3. All nurses must carry out comprehensive, systematic nursing assessments that take account of relevant physical, social, cultural, psychological, spiritual, genetic and environmental factors, in partnership with service users and others through interaction, observation and measurement.

10. All nurses must evaluate their care to improve clinical decision-making, quality and outcomes, using a range of methods, amending the plan of care, where necessary, and communicating changes to others.

NMC Essential Skills Clusters

This chapter will address the following ESCs:

Cluster: Organisational aspects of care

9. People can trust the newly registered graduate nurse to treat them as partners and work with them to make a holistic and systematic assessment of their needs: to develop a personalised plan that is based on mutual understanding and respect for their individual situation promoting health and wellbeing, minimising risk of harm and promoting their safety at all times.

By the first progression point:

1. Responds appropriately when faced with an emergency or a sudden deterioration in a person's physical or psychological condition (for example, abnormal vital signs, collapse, cardiac arrest, self-harm, extremely challenging behaviour, attempted suicide), including seeking help from an appropriate person.

Chapter 4

> *By the second progression point:*
> 8. Collects and interprets routine data, under supervision, related to the assessment and planning of care from a variety of sources.
>
> **Cluster: Nutrition and fluid management**
> 28. People can trust the newly registered graduate nurse to assess and monitor their nutritional status and, in partnership, formulate an effective plan of care.
>
> *By the second progression point:*
> 1. Takes and records accurate measurements of weight, height, length, BMI and other appropriate measures of nutritional status.

Chapter aims

After reading this chapter you should be able to:

- understand the purpose of assessment tools;
- identify the knowledge and skills needed to use assessment and screening tools and list some potential problems;
- understand a range of assessment tools, such as the Malnutrition Universal Screening Tool (MUST), Waterlow pressure ulcer prevention scoring system and the National Early Warning System (NEWS) score;
- identify how to utilise information gained from patient assessment to achieve a nursing diagnosis and a plan of care.

Introduction

Scenario: Collaborative use of a falls assessment tool

Rob was in the second year of his nurse preparation programme and his placement was with the Intermediate Care Team. He noticed that many different professions, such as occupational therapists, physiotherapists and nurses, worked alongside each other in this area. This was particularly evident with the falls assessment tool where the nurses completed one side relating to the patient's presenting history, social background, biographical information and nursing observations and the therapists completed mobility and independence assessment elements. The resultant document was then integrated with the medical assessment, enabling a multidisciplinary plan of care to be generated.

Rob noted in his reflective diary the advantages of collaborative practice enacted in this way, reducing repetition for the patient and subjective judgement based on their particular profession's take on the situation. The falls assessment tool also triggered certain actions which needed to be followed up. Rob thought this could be especially useful for less experienced professionals like himself.

It is important for students to gain an understanding of the relevance of generic assessment and screening tools and how to apply them so as to be able to assess patient needs accurately. Screening tools offer an important basis for planning care interventions. As the case study above highlights, they can be used collaboratively and also offer important trigger points to ensure that further actions are commenced, as appropriate. The information collected by screening tools is also useful for compiling audit data to identify the effectiveness of care. It is important that you understand the purpose and usefulness of a variety of screening tools to aid your patient assessment and care planning. This chapter will clarify the purpose of assessment tools as well as identify some potential problems with their use. It will introduce the MUST, Waterlow and NEWS screening tools and identify how collated information is used to make a nursing diagnosis. The activities offered throughout the chapter will help you to reflect on your own knowledge and skills as well as make use of some of the screening tools with a case study. You will be invited to apply some of the principles to your own practice experience.

The purpose of assessment tools

The purpose of assessment tools is to enable you to carry out an effective assessment. Barrett et al. (2012) state that assessment tools can be categorised by what they do:

- health screening and diagnosis – identifying the problem and its severity, for example the Amsterdam Preoperative Anxiety and Information scale (Pritchard, 2009);
- descriptive – describing the problem but not necessarily directing action, for example the Abbey pain-rating scale (Chapman, 2010);
- predictive – identifying the potential for problems to develop, for example the Multi-dimensional Falls assessment (Lyons et al., 2005).

What assessment tools do is offer a way to map the problem, or consider potential problems, in terms that can be easily communicated to other professionals. The negative aspect of this is that the terminology and process may not always be comprehensible to patients and therefore can exclude them from the process. Completing Activity 4.1 will help you to identify your knowledge about the range of assessment tools that are used in practice and their purpose.

Activity 4.1 — Critical thinking

Make a list of the assessment tools that you have seen used in your placements. Now consider:

- What was their purpose?
- Were other professionals involved in their use and if so, how?
- Were there any problems with using the tool?
- How was the patient involved?

As this activity is based on your experience, there is no outline answer at the end of the chapter.

You might have included some of the more commonly used assessment tools in your list, such as pressure ulcer scoring systems, pain assessment scales and the mini-mental score. You might have identified specific problems with patient involvement, such as the use of jargon, patient anxiety, cognitive ability and memory. It is also important to remember that assessment tools are only as good as the knowledge and expertise of the person using them. The National Institute for Health and Care Excellence (NICE) has developed a range of guidelines which underpin and inform many assessment tools (**www.nice.org.uk**). The next section explains in more detail the importance of knowledge and skills for using assessment tools.

Knowledge and skills needed to use assessment tools

An assessment tool used inaccurately can put patients at risk because you may over- or underestimate their risk of a particular problem or make inappropriate use of resources. It is important to ensure that you have the knowledge to use the tool and to continue to develop this with a diversity of patients, so that you can develop your skills and competence. Key aspects that need to be considered before using assessment tools are:

- knowledge of the tool – what is the purpose of using the tool and how relevant and suitable is it to the patient situation?
- knowledge and understanding of the patient's presenting problem and the reason for using the tool to assess this;
- communication – understanding how to gain information and explain what you are doing;
- obtaining data – understanding how to use the tool;
- recording data and information – understanding how to record the results accurately;
- evaluation of data and information – being able to analyse the results;
- linking results to diagnosis and care planning – being able to think critically about the results and analyse what to do next.

Consider the following case study and then complete Activity 4.2 in order to apply these principles.

Case study: Assessing pressure area risk

Niamh was working in a community placement with the district nurses in the first year of her preparation programme. They had a patient, Gladys, who was bed-bound. Niamh's mentor Mandy explained that they needed to assess Gladys' pressure area risk and asked Niamh whether she knew how to do this. Niamh replied that she had used the pressure risk assessment tool in hospital but was not sure if it was different in a community setting. Mandy showed Niamh how the pressure risk assessment tool was used in the community and then told her to have a go at assessing Gladys' needs. They discussed the results, which showed that Gladys was at high risk and needed specialist equipment.

Activity 4.2 — Critical thinking

Now you have read the case study see if you can answer the questions below:

- What questions does Niamh need to address before using the tool?
- What should she communicate to the patient?
- How should she record the results?
- What might she need to consider within her analysis of the results?

An outline answer is given at the end of the chapter.

When using an assessment tool it is important to explain as fully as possible to the patient what the tool is and why it is being used, to ensure patient consent. This is why you need to understand how the tool works and what you hope to achieve in using it, in order to give an accurate description. Therefore you need to address the following aspects when preparing to use an assessment tool so that you can justify what you are doing with the patient and communicate this to other professionals who may also be involved in the patient's care. Your explanation should include:

- the aim and objective of using the assessment tool;
- the benefits and limitations of the assessment tool;
- showing you have ensured that the information gathered is accurate;
- what you plan to do with the information gathered;
- any actions that have been triggered from using the assessment tool (think about possible nursing interventions and also whether you need to involve other people).

Being clear about why you are using a particular tool and what you hope to achieve provides justification for your actions and the opportunity for you to reflect on what you have learned from this instance of using the tool. This helps to develop your knowledge and skills further. Completing Activity 4.3 can help you to think about what you have learned from using assessment tools.

Activity 4.3 — Reflection

Think about an assessment tool you have used a number of times. Now consider the different situations you have used this tool in. What was similar and what was different? Were there any problems and how did you solve them? What do you think you have learned?

As this activity is based on your experience, there is no answer at the end of the chapter.

You might have considered your use of pain assessment tools. You might have identified how variable the results could be because of subjective scoring and interpretation and difficulty with determining action. You might have learned that you needed to integrate the information from the assessment tool with other information available to you so that you can make informed decisions about care planning.

Potential problems

Some potential problems of using assessment tools are that you can become overly reliant on them and therefore do not take sufficient note of the variety of evidence, of which they are only a part (Barrett et al., 2012). Mistakes can result from this and put the patient at risk. Equally, assessment tools may not be culturally sensitive and therefore may miss out important aspects, for example diet content. Continuously relying on assessment tools may also be deskilling because you use your clinical assessment skills less (Barrett et al., 2012). In order to provide holistic care it is important that you use your clinical observation skills and therapeutic communication to involve patients in your application of relevant assessment tools for their care. If you do not involve patients, how do you know what they are experiencing? Completing Activity 4.4 will help you to consider the relevance of clinical assessment skills for holistic assessment.

Activity 4.4 *Reflection*

List the clinical assessment skills that are important for developing holistic care. How could you develop these further? How could you increase patient involvement and ensure you are integrating the 6Cs?

An outline answer is given at the end of the chapter.

Making sure that you continue to develop all your assessment skills will help you to avoid some of the potential problems identified above. We proceed now to consider some selected assessment tools and how to use them.

Malnutrition Universal Screening Tool

The MUST is used to identify those who are malnourished, or at risk of becoming malnourished (Holmes, 2010). It assesses body mass index (BMI) through height and weight measurements, establishes the percentage of unintentional weight loss according to tables provided and scores subjective criteria such as the effects of acute disease, adding all these together to identify the overall risk (Malnutrition Advisory Group, reviewed 2012). The MUST tool and explanatory information can be viewed at the British Association for Parenteral and Enteral Nutrition website (**www.bapen.org.uk**). Holmes (2010) emphasises that the MUST tool should be used in conjunction with clinical assessment information so that a nutritional support plan can be commenced and evaluated over time. Nutritional health is important for the body's ability to fight infection and for growth and repair (Rushforth, 2009). NICE (2006) recommends that screening should be repeated in those cases where patients are deemed to be vulnerable (**www.nice.org.uk/CG32**). Such patients include those with:

- BMI <18.5;
- unintentional weight loss >10%;
- decreased absorptive capacity;
- increased nutritional requirement, e.g. burns or other large wounds such as abdominal surgery.

Case study: Simon's ulcerative colitis flare-up

Simon was 19 years old and due to start university. He had been diagnosed with ulcerative colitis in his early teens. As he prepared to go to university his symptoms of diarrhoea, abdominal cramps and general malaise worsened and he started to lose weight. On his way to meet a friend he collapsed and was taken to hospital. Following investigations in accident and emergency he was diagnosed with an acute exacerbation of ulcerative colitis and admitted to the gastrointestinal ward. The student nurse, Geena, who was admitting Simon completed the MUST score and noted that his BMI was 19, but that his weight loss was less than 5% over the last 3 months. This gave Simon a MUST score of 1, which meant he was at medium risk of malnutrition. Geena documented Simon's MUST score and relayed the result to her mentor, Peter. Peter explained that as Simon was at medium risk of malnutrition they would write that his nutritional intake was to be observed in the care plan, and that Simon was to be rescreened with the MUST tool in 3 days' time. Geena asked why they were not referring Simon to the dietician now. Peter explained that, as Simon was deemed to be medium risk, the objective was to see what Simon ate and if there was anything interfering with his food intake in order to make a considered judgement.

Over the next day it was noted that cramping pain was interfering with Simon eating. His pain relief was adjusted and as his medication to counteract the ulcerative colitis symptoms took effect, Simon began to eat more regularly. His repeat MUST screen indicated that Simon was now low risk and he was discharged home.

In Simon's case study you will have noted that his absorptive capacity has been reduced by the flare-up of his ulcerative colitis, putting him at medium risk of malnutrition despite his age. Completing Activity 4.5 will help you to identify some other patient situations where using the MUST tool would be indicated.

Activity 4.5 — Critical thinking

Make a list of patient problems correlated with the warning signs described above. What would alert you?

An outline answer is given at the end of the chapter.

In practice you may find that you will be using a number of assessment tools concurrently, especially with very sick patients. The next tool we will consider is the Waterlow pressure ulcer scoring system, which draws on some of the results from the MUST score.

Chapter 4

Waterlow pressure ulcer scoring system

The Waterlow pressure ulcer scoring system was developed by Judy Waterlow in 1985. She recognised the economic and human cost of pressure ulcers and has continued to revise and update the scoring system to include recent research (Waterlow, 2008). The scoring system provides categories which are scored according to the patient's presentation. The scores are then added together to identify the overall risk. The categories include:

- BMI;
- visual assessment of skin type;
- age and sex (gender);
- malnutrition screening;
- continence;
- mobility;
- special risks, such as surgery, trauma, disease effects and neurological deficits.

The overall risk is defined as at risk, high risk or very high risk, and a range of pressure-reducing aids and nursing care options is proposed (Waterlow, 2008). The latest Waterlow scoring system can be viewed at **www.judy-waterlow.co.uk** and you can download a useful quick guide. Completing Activity 4.6 will help you to identify the local version used in your practice area.

Activity 4.6 *Critical thinking*

Look at the quick guide in the Waterlow website (link given above). Now consider the pressure scoring system you have seen used in your practice, or look for one on your next placement. Are there any differences and if so, what might be the reasons? What does the local policy say?

As this activity is based on your experience and practice area, there is no answer at the end of the chapter.

Local policy takes account of research, national guidelines and other relevant assessment tools such as wound assessment. It is important that you inform yourself of local policies and guidelines in order to be able to evaluate critically your use of assessment tools and their effectiveness. Local policies are developed through practitioner feedback as well as research and national guidelines. We now proceed to consider the NEWS scoring system.

National Early Warning Score

There have been a number of early warning systems used in the care of acutely ill patients. The multiplicity of such systems used in healthcare institutions led to the development of a National

Standard because of differences in local systems and language. The NEWS score was developed to provide acute care teams with a system that enabled a timely response to acutely ill patients. Early detection and a competent, timely clinical response are the key determinants of the outcome for people who are acutely ill. The NEWS assessment tool was developed as a standardised scoring system to warn of physiological changes in the condition of patients who were very unwell, so that timely interventions could be implemented (Royal College of Physicians, 2012). NICE (2007) had previously recommended that acutely ill patients needed to be monitored more closely to identify deterioration in the acute hospital setting (**www.nice.org.uk/CG50**). The NEWS assessment tool integrates vital signs (temperature, pulse, respiration, blood pressure) with assessed levels of consciousness directing actions and appropriate intervals for re-evaluation so that deterioration in a patient can be identified and monitored. The specialised observation chart uses colours to denote when observation results are entering danger trigger zones. You will see these used in acute settings such as surgical and medical wards as well as intensive care and accident and emergency. When you next have an acute placement, examine the observation charts used and ask practitioners how they use them.

Of course many other assessment tools are available, such as falls, pain, anxiety, informational needs, self-esteem and body image, sedation scores and wound assessment, and different variations are also used. We have only focused on three of the most widely used assessment tools here. These are all applicable to the following case study.

Case study: Mr Barry's biliary stent

Mr Barry is a 70-year-old man who has liver cancer. He has become more jaundiced and unwell. Although his condition is terminal, there are palliation procedures which can help him. One of these is a biliary stent insertion which will help relieve pressure in the biliary duct and reduce the jaundice by allowing the bile to drain into the small bowel again, for a while. Mr Barry has lost considerable weight in the last month as he has lost his appetite and has felt quite nauseous. On admission his BMI is less than 18.5 and his skin is noted to be dry and warm. His vital signs are temperature 37.8°C, pulse 100bpm, respirations 15 breaths/minute, blood pressure 130/85mmHg. His urine output is 70ml/hour. The biliary stent procedure is undertaken in the radiology department, requiring Mr Barry to lie on a hard X-ray table for up to three hours. As it is a painful procedure Mr Barry is given pre-emptive analgesia of morphine and the sedative midazolam. The procedure is carried out successfully and Mr Barry returns to the ward after three hours. The next day his temperature starts to rise and over the next few days his condition deteriorates. His temperature is now 40.1°C, his pulse is 50bpm, respirations are 24 breaths/minute, blood pressure is 200/110mmHg and his urine output has fallen to 20ml/hour. Mr Barry is sometimes delirious. Blood cultures confirm that Mr Barry has septicaemia. He is moved to a high dependency unit for further monitoring. Intravenous antibiotics are started and Mr Barry gradually improves. After a week he is well enough to move out of the high dependency unit. However it is noted that he has developed a sacral pressure sore.

Read the above case study again and then use the assessment tools (Waterlow, MUST and NEWS) discussed earlier to complete Activity 4.7.

Activity 4.7 — Critical thinking

After reading the case study, use each of the Waterlow, MUST and NEWS assessment tools in turn and try to complete the tool you have chosen using the information provided. Now consider the following questions:

- What are the benefits and limitations of this tool in relation to the case study?
- What are the issues of using this tool with the patient case, e.g. do you have all the information you need or is some missing and, if so, how will you find it?
- What skills do you need?
- What actions are triggered by the use of the tool with the patient case?
- Who else might you need to involve?

An outline answer is given at the end of the chapter.

As you will have noted, the assessment tools all come to different conclusions. You need to analyse these conclusions and identify your nursing diagnosis of the situation. This is considered more in the next section.

Relationship of screening tools to making a nursing diagnosis

Screening tools help to identify the problems the patient has. The information provided by the assessment tool is analysed by practitioners to determine what to do next. Part of this analysis process is making a nursing diagnosis based on the results obtained, to direct further action and nursing interventions. Making a nursing diagnosis is what practitioners do when they are interacting with patients, for example, identifying whether a patient is anxious or in pain. It is important to be able to communicate what the nursing diagnosis is to the patient and to other professionals so that they can understand why you are following a particular course of action. The case study of Erica illustrates how this is done.

Case study: Making a nursing diagnosis of infection

*Erica was a 58-year-old woman who was having her leg ulcers redressed by the community nurse, Alicia. Alicia used a wound assessment chart to assess the progress of Erica's leg ulcers. Wound assessment charts vary between organisations, but commonly consider the dimensions of the wound, the appearance of the wound bed and surrounding skin, any exudate or bleeding, level of pain and location of the wound to be entered on the human diagram (Dougherty and Lister, 2011). (An example of a wound assessment chart can be found at the following link: **http://emedia.wounds-uk.com/woundcare/downloads/time_assessment_tool.pdf**.) When completing the assessment, Alicia noted that Erica seemed to be experiencing increasing*

> *discomfort. She examined Erica's leg ulcers and noted an increase in exudate and that the wound bed seemed to be showing signs of infection. Alicia made a nursing diagnosis of wound infection and altered the dressing regime. She explained to Erica why she was doing this. She also documented the change and her reasoning for this and communicated the change to Erica's GP.*

The case study highlights that nurses make decisions about nursing interventions. These are based on the information gleaned from patients in a variety of ways. Being able to make a nursing diagnosis is important because you need to justify the changes that you make. We will look at how to make a nursing diagnosis in greater detail in Chapter 5. Next we consider how screening tools contribute to audit.

Screening tools and audit

Screening tools are used within audit procedures because they provide consistent assessment of a phenomenon. For example, pressure sore prevalence audits are recommended to be undertaken regularly to benchmark the quality of patient care (Defloor et al., 2005). Audit collects and measures available information with the purpose of measuring care against evidence-based benchmarks (Barker, 2013). The European Pressure Ulcer Advisory Panel classification system differentiates between other wounds and pressure sores, helping practitioners to make this distinction in a systematic way (Defloor et al., 2005). Completing Activity 4.8 will help you to identify the link between other assessment tools and audit.

> **Activity 4.8** *Critical thinking*
>
> Make a list of any clinical audits you have seen completed in practice, or if you have not seen any, ask your mentor which audits are carried out in your placement area. What information is collected and what tools are used to collect it? How do the results inform practice?
>
> *An outline answer is given at the end of the chapter.*

You might like to explore the relevance of audit further by reading Ellis's (2013) evidence-based practice book (full reference at the end of this chapter under further reading). Accurate assessment and interpretation of information are important to manage clinical effectiveness and promote high quality patient care.

Conclusion

Assessment tools are useful for gaining information about problems, or potential problems, which patients may experience as well as playing an important part in auditing the quality of care. They use a systematic approach and provide suggested further action which is especially helpful to less experienced practitioners. Nevertheless, they should not take the place of other forms of clinical assessment such as observing and talking to patients to identify what they need.

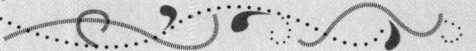

Chapter summary

This chapter has examined the importance and relevance of assessment tools to patient assessment. The benefits and limitations of using assessment tools have been considered. Three of the most commonly used assessment tools – MUST, Waterlow and NEWS – have been referred to. It is important to recognise that the assessment tool is only as effective as the knowledge and skill of the person using it. Therefore a range of activities to develop your knowledge and skills have been integrated into the chapter. Reflection on their continuing development will help you to become more effective and accurate in your patient assessments and to make a nursing diagnosis.

Activities: brief outline answers

Activity 4.2 Critical thinking [page 55]

Niamh needs to find out what is wrong with Gladys in order to determine the suitability of the assessment tool and how to interpret the results. She will also need to check with her mentor whether her understanding of the tool, gained from using it in the hospital setting, is appropriate for the community setting before starting to use it with Gladys. Niamh will need to explain to Gladys what she intends to do and why and gain her consent. She will then need to use the assessment tool prompts to gather the data, record the results on the tool paperwork and then interpret the results, again explaining these to Gladys and what the next actions are. She will need to record these in the nursing notes. Lastly she will need to evaluate her use of the tool reflectively with her mentor in order to inform her future practice.

Activity 4.4 Reflection [page 56]

Clinical assessment skills include questioning techniques and attentive listening (return to Chapter 3 to review these), observation and analytical thinking. Analytical thinking in particular aims to integrate all the assessments undertaken by a variety of professionals so that appropriate interventions can be commenced. You could develop your clinical assessment skills further by practising them regularly with each patient you encounter and making sure you are always taking a complete view rather than concentrating on a narrow fragment. You could involve patients more by asking them about their experience and offering information and explanation. You can integrate the 6Cs through developing your competence and through communicating appropriately to find out the patient's perspective. In this way you can also demonstrate your commitment and care.

Activity 4.5 Critical thinking [page 57]

Problems that could result in a BMI of <18.5 include eating disorders such as anorexia nervosa and bulimia, mental illness such as depression and physical illnesses such as cancer, particularly when patients are having chemo- or radiotherapy and when they are in the palliative stages. Sudden unexplained weight loss is often a sign of cancer. In the elderly it may be because they do not have an appetite for a variety of reasons, or have swallowing difficulties. Decreased absorptive capacity problems include Crohn's disease and ulcerative colitis and certain types of bowel surgery. Increased nutritional requirements are exerted by large wounds such as extensive pressure ulcers and burns and also by prolonged infection. Aspects that might alert you could include:

- mood and mental state;
- picking at food;
- lack of interest in appearance or hygiene;
- withdrawal from communication;
- vomiting and diarrhoea;
- pain.

Activity 4.7 Critical thinking [page 60]

Using the MUST tool with Mr Barry's case you will have identified that he is at high risk of malnutrition. You do not know the percentage of weight he has lost but take into account his subjective view that it is considerable. You consider the benefits of using the MUST tool as identifying Mr Barry's nutritional risk, but its limitation is that it is based on a cognitively aware patient. The skills you need for using the tool are knowledge of how to use it and professional judgement of the patient problem and likely effects. The action triggered by the MUST tool is nutritional support. You would involve the dietician to advise.

Using the Waterlow score with Mr Barry's case, you will have identified that he is at high risk to very high risk of developing a pressure sore. You do not know the effect of lying on a hard X-ray table or how much weight he has lost. You consider the benefit of using this scoring system as identifying Mr Barry's pressure risk but note its limitations in that it is based on your subjective interpretation as well as giving a tendency to overestimate. The skills you need to use the tool are observational and analytical. The main issue of using this tool with this patient case is his changing condition and needs. The actions triggered are to provide pressure-relieving aids, ensure appropriate manual handling techniques are used and to grade the pressure sore and apply dressing as per local policy. For this you might involve the local tissue viability nurse.

Using the NEWS assessment tool, you would have identified that Mr Barry's vital signs and level of consciousness have triggered the need for more frequent recording of observations and for review of Mr Barry by the intensive care outreach team. You consider the benefits of using this assessment tool as alerting you to Mr Barry's deterioration and of involving relevant other professionals at an early stage. You consider the limitations of the tool as having areas where the patient is in between and this can lead to uncertainty of what to do. The skills needed to use this tool are being able to carry out accurate nursing observations and understanding the significance of these observations. The actions triggered are more frequent nursing observations and involvement of the outreach team, and notifying the radiology team who carried out the biliary stenting procedure.

Activity 4.8 Critical thinking [page 61]

The type of audits carried out in practice are likely to include mortality rates following medical intervention, resuscitation outcomes, pressure ulcer prevalence, infection rates and record keeping. What these have in common is that an assessment tool for finding out the information will be used. Assessment is therefore also important for practice in order to continue practice development.

Further reading

Barrett, D, Wilson, B and Woollands, A (2012) *Care Planning: A Guide for Nurses*, 2nd edn. Harlow: Pearson Education.

This book has a useful section on the advantages and disadvantages of assessment tools and will help you to set their use within the wider context of care planning.

Ellis, P (2013) *Evidence-Based Practice in Nursing*, 2nd edn. London: SAGE Publications.

This book has a clear section on the importance of audit and will help inform your thinking about this.

Chapter 4

Useful websites

www.bapen.org.uk
This website gives information about the MUST score.

www.judy-waterlow.co.uk
This website identifies how to use the Waterlow scoring system.

www.nice.org.uk
This website offers information on NICE guidelines.

www.nice.org.uk/CG32
This link takes you to the page for Clinical Guideline 32, which offers specific information on nutritional assessment.

www.nice.org.uk/CG50
This link takes you to the page for Clinical Guideline 50, which gives specific information on the assessment of deterioration in acutely ill adults.

Chapter 5
Nursing diagnosis

Lioba Howatson-Jones

> **NMC Standards for Pre-registration Nursing Education**
>
> This chapter will address the following competencies:
>
> **Domain 3: Nursing practice and decision-making**
> 1. All nurses must use up-to-date knowledge and evidence to assess, plan, deliver and evaluate care, communicate findings, influence change and promote health and best practice. They must make person-centred, evidence-based judgements and decisions, in partnership with others involved in the care process, to ensure high-quality care. They must be able to recognise when the complexity of clinical decisions requires specialist knowledge and expertise, and consult or refer accordingly.
> 4. All nurses must ascertain and respond to the physical, social and psychological needs of people, groups and communities. They must then plan, deliver and evaluate safe, competent, person-centred care in partnership with them, paying special attention to changing health needs during different life stages, including progressive illness and death, loss and bereavement.
>
> **Domain 4: Leadership, management and team working**
> 3. All nurses must be able to identify priorities and manage time and resources effectively to ensure the quality of care is maintained or enhanced.

> **NMC Essential Skills Clusters**
>
> This chapter will address the following ESCs:
>
> **Cluster: Organisational aspects of care**
> 14. People can trust the newly registered graduate nurse to be an autonomous and confident member of the multidisciplinary or multiagency team and to inspire confidence in others.
>
> *By the first progression point:*
> 1. Works within the code (Nursing and Midwifery Council, 2008, 2015) and adheres to the *Guidance on Professional Conduct for Nursing and Midwifery Students* (Nursing and Midwifery Council, 2010).

Chapter 5

> *continued ...*
> *By the second progression point:*
> 5. Communicates with colleagues verbally, face to face and by telephone, and in writing and electronically in a way that the meaning is clear, and checks that the communication has been fully understood.
> 16. People can trust the newly registered graduate nurse to safely lead, co-ordinate and manage care.

> **Chapter aims**
>
> After reading this chapter you should be able to:
>
> - define what is meant by nursing diagnosis;
> - explain the history and development of nursing diagnosis;
> - identify how nursing diagnosis relates to the patient assessment process;
> - consider some of the potential benefits and problems of nursing diagnosis for the patient and nurse as well as some of the advantages and disadvantages;
> - develop a nursing diagnosis from a patient assessment.

Introduction

Nursing diagnosis is a process in which nurses establish nursing priorities from their communication and interaction with patients. This chapter will explain what a nursing diagnosis is and how you can develop one. It will also identify some of the advantages and disadvantages of a nursing diagnosis and what this means for the patient and the nurse.

What is meant by nursing diagnosis?

Wilkinson and Ahern (2009) define a nursing diagnosis as:

> *a concise label that describes patient conditions observed in practice. These conditions may be actual or potential problems or wellness diagnoses.*
> (Wilkinson and Ahern, 2009, p6)

The important point here is that a nursing diagnosis requires accurate description of the main characteristics. However, this presents problems because terminology varies between different professions and professionals and therefore standardisation of terms helps to ensure consistency (Carpenito-Moyet, 2013). For example, a doctor might talk about hypoglycaemia whereas a nurse may describe this as low blood sugar. Nurses do try to demystify medical terminology to help patients to understand what they have been told, but what Carpenito-Moyet (2013) is suggesting is that nurses also need to be consistent in the terminology they use. The following case study identifies how a nursing diagnosis is established.

Case study: Su's informational needs

Su is a 53-year-old woman who has recently had her first breast-screening appointment. She is recalled to the clinic for further imaging due to an abnormality being found. Su is very nervous and concerned. She has further radiological images taken followed by a breast biopsy and sees the breast physician for the results a week later. Su is told that she has a fibroadenoma – a benign tumour. As it is small, nothing further needs to be done. Su goes home relieved. However, when talking it over with her husband, Su starts to worry. The word 'tumour' sticks in her mind. Su equates the word 'tumour' with cancer. Su begins to find it difficult to sleep and eat and is anxious most of the time. She is worried that the benign tumour may develop into a cancerous one. She goes to see the nurse at her GP surgery. Hayley, the nurse, makes a nursing diagnosis of informational need. Hayley explains to Su that a fibroadenoma is a small knot of fibrous and glandular cells. These cells are a normal component of breast tissue but have multiplied too much. The breast biopsy has confirmed the medical diagnosis, that the cells are benign. 'Benign' means that the cells will not become cancerous and spread, but will stay in their present location. Removal of the lump is only indicated if the fibroadenoma is particularly large. Hayley advises Su to become familiar with the feel of the lump so she can notice and act on any changes. In this way Su can regain some control. After seeing Hayley, Su feels much better. She remembers that the breast physician did explain some of this to her, but she was too agitated at the time to take it in. Su also asks her husband to become familiar with the feel and shape of her breast and help to alert her to any change he may notice.

The case study above illustrates how the medical diagnosis of a benign fibroadenoma has left Su with further informational needs. This is partly because Su was too anxious to take in what was being said by the doctor, but also because she did not understand the medical jargon which the breast physician used. Hayley has listened to Su's concerns and from this has established a nursing diagnosis of unmet need for information. The case study shows that, although medical and nursing diagnoses may be related, they often have differing foci and emphasis. The focus of the medical diagnosis is physiological; the focus of the nursing diagnosis in this case is the psychological impact of the physiological problem. Carpenito-Moyet (2013) asserts that nurses need to establish a classification system that describes not only the patient problem, but also patient responses, which are considered when making a nursing diagnosis. The key aspects of a nursing diagnosis are:

- defining the nursing problem – for example, the person is unable to get out of bed;
- describing the characteristics of that problem using information from the patient and from objective assessment such as the use of an assessment tool – for example, the patient says she cannot stand without support; a recent falls assessment identifies that she cannot balance due to right-sided leg weakness following a cerebrovascular accident;
- considering other relevant factors – for example, level of visual acuity;
- considering different diagnoses for best fit – for example, pain or arthritis causing immobility;
- identifying what you hope to achieve – for example, for the patient to be able to get out of bed as independently as possible (Wilkinson and Ahern, 2009).

Nevertheless, trying to standardise terms should not distract nurses from clarifying information given to patients. Nursing diagnosis and medical diagnosis are different because the nursing emphasis is on a holistic assessment of the patient which considers psychological as well as physical concerns (Barrett et al., 2012).

What a nursing diagnosis is not, is simply stating a patient problem, such as 'cannot mobilise'. The problem needs to be defined. In contrast, a medical diagnosis will focus on a health deficit, such as rectal bleeding, for example, which is established by the medical practitioner. Nursing diagnoses try to involve and include patients by taking account of their experience and how this feels for them. Completing Activity 5.1 will help you to reflect on your understanding of a nursing diagnosis.

> **Activity 5.1** *Reflection*
>
> Think about your last placement and the patients you cared for. How did you formulate their problems and needs? How did your mentor describe patient problems and needs? How did other professionals such as doctors and therapists describe patient problems and needs?
>
> Now compare and contrast how the patient formulated their problems and needs. Were there any differences and how could you reconcile them?
>
> *As this activity is based on your experience, there is a limited answer at the end of the chapter.*

You may have identified that you carry out the instructions of others without always knowing how they are framing the nursing diagnosis. You may have thought about some of the descriptors used for patient problems, such as immobile, incontinent, unable to self-care. These are however rather vague and could be more precise in order to help practitioners think about what to do. Dougherty and Lister (2011) make the point that patient problems and nursing diagnoses may not always be phrased the same because other disciplines may not always see the problem in the same way. This is why it is important for nurses to take a holistic view in order to develop a nursing diagnosis which takes into account the involvement of other disciplines as well as the patient. In the next section we consider how and why nursing diagnoses started to be used.

The history and development of nursing diagnosis

The history of nursing diagnosis grew out of the frustration of nurses with a biomedical view of illness and caring which focused on the disease and not the person and which ignored nurses' observations of patient responses. Nursing diagnosis is not a new concept. Florence Nightingale was commenting over a hundred years ago on the need for hospitals to keep records that enabled comparisons to be made on the effectiveness of care (Nightingale, 1859, cited by Weir-Hughes, 2007, p35). Systematic methods of planning and evaluating patient care were introduced globally into nursing programmes of learning and practice in the 1970s (Gordon, 1994). In the USA nursing diagnoses began to be used in the 1950s and were gradually amalgamated into nursing practice through the efforts of first the American Nurses Association and then through further definition by the North American Nursing Diagnosis Association (NANDA) as part of the nursing process (Carpenito-Moyet, 2013) (there will be further discussion of the nursing process in a later section). Around the same time Carper (1978) was developing her theories of nursing knowledge as being different from medical knowledge and these have also informed the process of developing a nursing diagnosis. These theories see patients as unique, with their own resources and strengths that need to be considered. NANDA has defined and characterised many of the nursing diagnoses that patients are likely to present with in a variety of settings (see **www.nanda.org**). Examples include anxiety, grieving, hopelessness, acute pain, risk for violence, impaired mobility, deficient fluid volume, nutrition imbalance and many more (Carpenito-Moyet, 2013). Nurses are becoming more empowered through defining what the nursing diagnosis is and this in turn is helping them to be clear in their definition of what nursing is. Completing Activity 5.2 will help you to understand this point.

Activity 5.2 — Reflection

Think about when you first considered nursing as a career. What did you think nursing was? What informed your definition? What do you think nursing is now? What has informed your conclusion?

An outline answer is given at the end of the chapter.

It is important for you to realise that you are contributing to the definition of nursing that others are experiencing and for you to be able to justify the choices of action you have made. This begins from your initial patient assessment. In your assessment and decision-making you are helping to develop nursing diagnoses further and thereby are also adding to the knowledge in nursing. We move on now to consider some of the advantages and disadvantages of using nursing diagnoses.

Advantages and disadvantages of nursing diagnoses

No nursing process should be undertaken without first reflecting upon whether it is fit for purpose and likely to achieve what you are aiming for. There will be more on the nursing process in the next section. While it is acknowledged that discipline expertise between nursing and medicine overlaps in areas of disease prevention, taking a history, diagnosing medical problems and seeking consultant advice, there are also many areas of difference, particularly in relation to nursing and medical definition and management of problems (Carpenito-Moyet, 2013). Like most processes, nursing diagnoses come with advantages and disadvantages.

cited by Weir-Hughes, 2007, p35). Systematic methods of planning and evaluating patient care were introduced globally into nursing programmes of learning and practice in the 1970s (Gordon, 1994). In the USA nursing diagnoses began to be used in the 1950s and were gradually amalgamated into nursing practice through the efforts of first the American Nurses Association and then through further definition by the North American Nursing Diagnosis Association (NANDA) as part of the nursing process (Carpenito-Moyet, 2013) (there will be further discussion of the nursing process in a later section). Around the same time Carper (1978) was developing her theories of nursing knowledge as being different from medical knowledge and these have also informed the process of developing a nursing diagnosis. These theories see patients as unique, with their own resources and strengths that need to be considered. NANDA has defined and characterised many of the nursing diagnoses that patients are likely to present with in a variety of settings (see **www.nanda.org**). Examples include anxiety, grieving, hopelessness, acute pain, risk for violence, impaired mobility, deficient fluid volume, nutrition imbalance and many more (Carpenito-Moyet, 2013). Nurses are becoming more empowered through defining what the nursing diagnosis is and this in turn is helping them to be clear in their definition of what nursing is. Completing Activity 5.2 will help you to understand this point.

Activity 5.2   Reflection

Think about when you first considered nursing as a career. What did you think nursing was? What informed your definition? What do you think nursing is now? What has informed your conclusion?

An outline answer is given at the end of the chapter.

It is important for you to realise that you are contributing to the definition of nursing that others are experiencing and for you to be able to justify the choices of action you have made. This begins from your initial patient assessment. In your assessment and decision-making you are helping to develop nursing diagnoses further and thereby are also adding to the knowledge in nursing. We move on now to consider some of the advantages and disadvantages of using nursing diagnoses.

Advantages and disadvantages of nursing diagnoses

No nursing process should be undertaken without first reflecting upon whether it is fit for purpose and likely to achieve what you are aiming for. There will be more on the nursing process in the next section. While it is acknowledged that discipline expertise between nursing and medicine overlaps in areas of disease prevention, taking a history, diagnosing medical problems and seeking consultant advice, there are also many areas of difference, particularly in relation to nursing and medical definition and management of problems (Carpenito-Moyet, 2013). Like most processes, nursing diagnoses come with advantages and disadvantages.

Advantages of nursing diagnoses

- They clearly define the problem – it is important to be able to communicate patient problems clearly to nurses and other healthcare practitioners.
- They focus on the patient you are dealing with rather than all patients – patients are unique and nursing diagnoses reflect this.
- They consider nursing priorities, which may differ from medical ones – they consider problems from other scientific viewpoints such as the social sciences.
- They direct specific nursing action and evaluation of that action – nursing diagnoses provide the basis on which care is planned and evaluated (Hinchliff et al., 2008).

Therefore, by clearly defining the problem and the actions which should follow, criteria are established by which to measure outcomes. This may be particularly beneficial for novice nurses and those new to practice.

However there are also some disadvantages of nursing diagnoses.

Disadvantages of nursing diagnoses

- The patient does not understand the nursing diagnosis – patients need to be included in discussion when the nursing diagnosis is being drawn up so that they can see how the nursing diagnosis is different from the medical diagnosis.
- The terminology may not be easily transferable to different healthcare systems.
- Nursing diagnosis-directed interventions can be prescriptive – the actions asked for dictate what should be done and may not allow other interpretation according to unique patient circumstance.
- Nursing judgements can become formulaic, restricting learning.
- Care is fragmented – nursing diagnoses give specific directions to nursing interventions which can deconstruct the act of nursing care to a task (Carpenito-Moyet, 2013).

Some of these disadvantages are avoidable when nurses are self-aware and do not try to impose their own values and understanding of the patient situation, or make judgements about the patient. We now proceed to consider how nursing diagnosis relates to the patient assessment process.

How nursing diagnosis relates to the patient assessment process

The nursing process is a systematic way of problem-solving which integrates assessment information with decisions made about care. It includes critically thinking about potential nursing interventions to develop a care strategy and then evaluating the outcomes of the care provided. The nursing process has been used for some time in the UK because it can help to articulate evidence-based nursing care (Dyson, 2004). Establishing the nursing diagnosis is a key part of the nursing process because it identifies what the nursing priorities are. The nursing process is cyclical and begins with patient assessment which, combined with communication with the patient, helps the nurse to develop the nursing diagnosis. This is an important leadership role for all nurses as they take the lead in nursing care for their patient(s).

Nurses use information obtained through patient assessment to make clinical judgements about the nursing care the patient needs. These clinical judgements are nursing diagnoses (Dougherty and Lister, 2011). This suggests that there is a definite process to making a nursing diagnosis and subsequent decisions about care. Carpenito-Moyet (2013) identifies that patients are the starting point in the experiences they describe, the signs and symptoms they display and their responses to medical interventions. Barrett et al. (2012) state that using a systematic nursing diagnosis enables problem reflection and finding solutions. These are important considerations when trying to identify possible nursing problems and from this a possible nursing diagnosis is made. Figure 5.1 shows the stages in the cycle which adds nursing diagnosis to the nursing process, as suggested by Barrett et al. (2012).

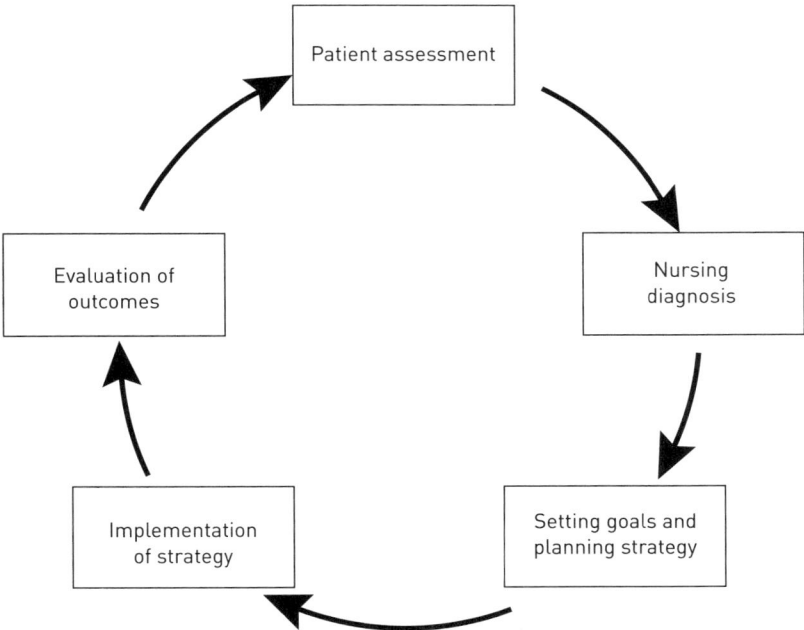

Figure 5.1: Nursing diagnosis as part of the nursing process

Because a systematic nursing diagnosis focuses not only on disease processes or treatment options but also on nursing priorities, the outcomes looked for by nurses may be different from those sought by medical practitioners (Welton and Halloran, 2005). Accurate documentation of the nursing diagnosis process and implementation of the nursing actions planned are important for continuing effective and safe patient care (Paans et al., 2011). The following case study illustrates how nursing diagnosis fits into the nursing process of assessment and care planning.

> **Case study: Diagnosing John's inability to cope**
>
> *John is a retired postman. He is married with two grown-up children, one of whom lives in New Zealand and the other has a high-powered job in London. John's wife died 6 months ago and he has lost interest in looking after himself. His GP has become concerned that John is depressed and has referred him to the mental health team. Gillian, the mental health nurse, visits John at home. She notices the dirty state of the house and unwashed cups and dishes in the kitchen. She also sees the stubble on John's chin and smells body odour. She asks John how he has been getting on and how things are since his wife died. John looks sad and starts to cry. Gillian remains silent, but places a hand on John's to offer comfort. Gillian gives John time by moving on to discuss his current medication regime prescribed by his GP. When John is more composed, Gillian asks how he has been managing to look after himself. John says he has no appetite and sits most days in front of the television for company. Gillian asks him whether he has had any bereavement counselling.*
>
> *Gillian makes a nursing diagnosis of inability to cope which she defines as John not being able to carry out normal activities and avoiding people. She plans with John what to do. She finds out that John belongs to a local church, although he has not been since his wife died. Gillian gains John's agreement for her to talk to the vicar to come and see him and organise some help with cooking and cleaning from the congregation. Gillian also arranges for a Cruse group member to come and speak to John. When Gillian visits John the following week he appears a bit more alert and interested. The visit of the Cruse group member has had a profound impact on him. He is talking about going to a group support session. Gillian sees this as regaining some ability to cope.*

The above case study illustrates how nurses can define nursing problems and find solutions working with patients. Gillian is clear about the problem, but does not try to impose solutions based on her own values; she works with activities and people associated with John. Nevertheless, this can sometimes also create problems when those people are not party to the meeting, but are called upon to contribute in some way. Therefore continuous evaluation of implementation strategies is important to check on their validity and effectiveness for patient care.

Potential benefits and problems of nursing diagnosis for the patient and nurse

One of the benefits of accurate nursing diagnosis is that it can help promote effective patient care and thereby potentially reduce the length of time that care is required (Weir-Hughes, 2007). What this means is that patients are able to return to their normal routines and leave care settings earlier because nurses focus on different outcomes to medicine (Welton and Halloran, 2005). In this way nurses are able to demonstrate systematically the contribution nursing makes to patient care in the way they think about patient problems. In the case study relating to John we have seen that he is able to recover partially through Gillian's nursing diagnosis, enabling her to plan potential strategies with John. The nursing process which incorporates nursing diagnosis as the next stage after patient assessment offers practitioners a chance to reflect and gives them directions for doing so, which is particularly helpful to the novice practitioner (Barrett et al., 2012).

Conversely, problems which may arise from such systematic thinking are that patients may feel they are being 'processed' rather than being viewed as individuals with unique needs. Gillian might have spent her first meeting with John completing paperwork instead and firing questions at him. This would have made John feel like he was being 'processed'. When nurses are reliant on a process it can also sometimes be difficult for them to think creatively and differently about their patient's problems and identify innovative solutions. Gillian identified one creative solution, John getting involved with his local church group again as well as a Cruse support group, as a foundation for developing interaction. Read the following case study and then complete Activity 5.3 afterwards in order to identify some other potential benefits and problems with establishing a nursing diagnosis.

Case study: Jon's spiritual needs

Jon is a 10-year-old boy with leukaemia. He has had radiotherapy and a bone marrow transplant, but these have been unsuccessful. He is now having chemotherapy, which he is finding very tiring. Jon's mother, Angie, is staying with him in the hospital where he has been admitted because his blood count is low. Angie is exhausted and finds it really difficult to talk to Jon about his illness as she knows his prognosis is poor and she cannot hide her distress from him. Jon knows his mother is distressed, but cannot talk to her about it because she shuts him out by talking about 'childish' things. Jon confides his concern for his mother to Maureen, an older nurse working in the children's cancer unit and someone whom Jon trusts. Jon says that he knows he is going to die and that everyone dies eventually anyway, so why hide from it? What he is finding hard is that no one seems to want to talk to him about it and they are always trying to 'jolly him along'. Jon has so many ideas and questions which he is looking to have answered. Maureen identifies that Jon has unmet spiritual needs. She sits down with him and asks him what he wants to know. Jon asks what will happen to him at the end and will he be in pain? Maureen tells him that he will become more and more tired and eventually slip into unconsciousness. Jon asks if this is like sleeping, but Maureen is careful to make the distinction between sleep and unconsciousness so that Jon is not concerned to go to sleep at night. She suggests Jon starts keeping a diary so that he can record his thoughts and feelings. Maureen says that this might help him when he finds the right time to talk with his mum, but in the meantime Maureen is happy to talk with him whenever she is working. Jon asks what will happen to his things when he dies and Maureen tells him they will be given to his mother. Jon thinks about this for a long time and then says that his diary can be a present to his mum.

Over the next week Jon writes and draws in his diary and at the end of the week Maureen finds Jon and Angie talking quietly. Angie later comes to find Maureen to thank her for helping her and Jon. She says that Jon's acceptance of his illness has helped to calm some of her own fears. The other nurses ask Maureen what she did as they have noticed a change in the relationship between Jon and his mother.

Jon gradually deteriorates and Maureen is now assigned to his care each time she is working. Jon dies at the end of the following week. Maureen gathers up his things and gives them to his mother, telling her that the diary was a special present from Jon to her.

> **Activity 5.3** — *Critical thinking*
>
> Read the case study about Jon again and identify the potential benefits of the nursing diagnosis for Jon, for Maureen and for other professionals. What might be the potential consequences for Jon's mother? Then consider any potential problems which the nursing diagnosis might create for the same group of people.
>
> Having read Jon's case study think about patients you have recently met on placement. Through reflection how would you develop a nursing diagnosis of their spiritual needs? Which of the 6Cs does this relate to?
>
> *An outline answer is given at the end of the chapter.*

Spirituality is often the section in patient assessment that is left blank or completed incorrectly in terms of focusing only on religious beliefs. However, spirituality is much more than this in terms of how people perceive themselves existing in the universe and have a sense of being (Clarke, 2013). Being able to explain to others the characteristics of the nursing diagnosis and how you are using it also includes risk-assessing it in terms of the potential benefits and problems. In the case study, Jon and Angie have benefited from Maureen's creative thinking. However, there are also risks attached because Maureen has only a snapshot view of their relationship and Jon's maturity of understanding. Maureen's good communication skills helped to support her development of the nursing diagnosis as well as its problem-solving, finding a solution and plan for implementation. The ward manager asked Maureen to give a talk to the new students starting on the ward about how to make a nursing diagnosis about spiritual need. Maureen relates the story of her experience to help illustrate how and why the nursing diagnosis of unmet spiritual need can help to plan useful interventions which can have profound consequences and outcomes. From having looked at some of the particular benefits and problems that establishing a nursing diagnosis can pose, you should now be ready to start to develop nursing diagnoses yourself from a patient assessment.

Developing a nursing diagnosis from a patient assessment

Carpenito-Moyet (2013) identifies a number of different categories of nursing diagnosis. These include:

- actual – the diagnosis is supported by the presence of major defining characteristics such as verbalisation of the inability to cope;
- risk – identifying vulnerability to the problem, such as risk of carer strain;
- possible diagnosis – there are cues for a possible problem but further information is needed to confirm this; for example, non-compliance might be an informed autonomous decision or might relate to lack of understanding;

- wellness – identifying the potential for being even better, such as managing health more effectively;
- syndrome diagnosis – a number of nursing diagnoses relate to a specific event; for example, domestic violence may give rise to a number of different nursing diagnoses but these all relate to a specific event;
- diagnostic cluster – these are nursing diagnoses that relate to particular patient group situations, such as standard post-procedure care, for example following an endoscopy.

In order to assess the patient you will need to collect and interpret information (return to Chapter 3 for more detail on this). This will include:

- medical history;
- history of the current problem;
- how the patient is feeling;
- patient understanding of the problem.

All of these contribute to you being able to establish a nursing diagnosis. You will also need to think about psychological, physiological, sociocultural, spiritual and environmental factors as well as the skills you need to deploy in relation to communication, analysis, creative thinking and problem-solving. Consider the following case study and then complete Activity 5.4.

Case study: Mabel's accident

Mabel is 56 years old and has learning difficulties. She lives in the community in a residential house. Mabel was crossing the road and got hit by a car which did not stop. Mabel was found unconscious by a cyclist who called an ambulance and stayed with her until it arrived.

Mabel wakes up in the ambulance, but remains groggy and confused. Her Glasgow coma score (GCS) is 13. She has a headache and vomits once before reaching the hospital. Mabel is medically diagnosed with a head injury and admitted to the trauma ward.

When admitted to the trauma ward Mabel becomes agitated by the strange environment and lashes out. She stays in the ward one night for observation and to receive anti-sickness medication and analgesia for her headache. When Mabel is discharged she is given head injury advice and told to come back if her symptoms worsen. This is repeated to the care worker who comes to collect Mabel.

Activity 5.4   Critical thinking

After reading the case study think about and list the different nursing diagnoses you can develop for Mabel. What categories do they fit with? What are the defining characteristics?

An outline answer is given at the end of the chapter.

You will have identified the possible nursing diagnoses as fitting into each of the categories described earlier. It might have been harder to think about the terms in which you wanted to describe them. Have a look at the diagnoses laid out in Carpenito-Moyet (2013), listed under 'Further reading' at the end of this chapter, to help you with this.

Conclusion

Nursing diagnoses offer a nursing perspective on the problems that patients present with and can be focused on just the nursing elements or in collaboration with other professionals. They articulate what expert nurses do all the time and therefore are especially useful for those who are less experienced in practice. Nursing diagnoses are systematic and the starting point for any subsequent care planning. Therefore they need to be accurately defined so that they are universally understood.

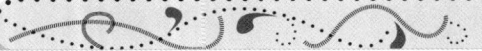

Chapter summary

This chapter has explained what nursing diagnosis is and offered some examples of different nursing diagnoses. It has clarified some of the advantages and disadvantages of using nursing diagnoses as well as some of the potential problems they may pose for the patient and the nurse. You have been challenged to begin to think about your definition of nursing in order to contribute to advancing the profession further. You have been invited through the activities to apply your critical thinking to the development of nursing diagnoses in different situations. They are the starting point for planning care and making decisions about care. This will be picked up again in Chapter 10.

Activities: brief outline answers

Activity 5.1 Reflection [page 68]

You might have formulated patients' problems and needs according to their medical diagnosis, what information was handed over to you and what patients said. Terminology is therefore likely to have varied. Your mentor is likely to have formulated patients' problems and needs in established nursing terms based on the patients' responses and observed behaviours. Doctors and therapists are likely to have formulated patients' problems and needs in precise terms based on medical terminology. The key difference with how patients are likely to formulate their problems are in the use of lay terms to describe their experiences, and in identifying how they are feeling rather than putting a diagnosis to the problem. Nevertheless, this is likely to vary depending on the problem and patient expertise.

Activity 5.2 Reflection [page 69]

You may have initially thought that nursing was about caring for people, although you could not really define this other than supporting patients who are feeling unwell by making them as comfortable as possible. You might also have identified nursing as giving medications. You could have been informed by the media and some of the programme dramas about nurses. You may also have based your definition on personal experience of being a patient. You are likely to realise now that nursing is based on the diagnoses that nurses make and which determine their nursing actions. While care is a key principle in any action taken by nurses, you need to be able to articulate your nursing diagnosis in order to explain your actions. What will have informed this conclusion is your placement experiences of seeing other nurses in action and being a novice nurse yourself. This is further informed by your learning theoretical elements such as accountability and the principles of the 6Cs. Nursing, therefore, is about recognising the uniqueness of each person and their individual needs and developing a nursing diagnosis which directs nursing actions to help individuals attain their health potential. As spirituality is a part of health, considering spiritual concerns is especially important for those who are dying to ensure the experience is as good as it can be in the circumstances.

Activity 5.3 Critical thinking [page 74]

You might have identified the benefits of this nursing diagnosis as making sure that Jon's needs are respected and acknowledged by him receiving honest answers to his questions. In addition the relationship between him and his mother is improved through the diary, stimulating discussion about his spiritual needs. The potential benefits for Jon's mother are also having a lasting memento from Jon, a reduction in her anxiety and of feeling supported. The benefits to Jon's nurse Maureen are that she is able to identify Jon's individual need in addition to that of his medical diagnosis of leukaemia and deterioration, and teach others how to do this, from her experiential learning. The benefits to other professionals are that they are aware of how Jon's spiritual needs are being considered. The potential problems you might have identified are the risk of further alienation between Jon and his mother and that the diary could increase her pain after his death through what Jon has written. The potential problem for the nurse is in accurately gauging Jon's mental maturity to be able to understand and deal with the truth of his dying. The problem for other professionals may be in understanding Maureen's reasoning processes. Documenting her reasoning using the standardised care plan and clear terms could be helpful to support other professionals' understanding. The most relevant core values from the 6Cs here are care and compassion.

Activity 5.4 Critical thinking [page 75]

You could have identified an actual diagnosis of a lack of understanding and communication issues. This would have been evident from the responses Mabel gave. You might also have identified a syndrome diagnosis of head injury which included the headache and nausea which Mabel was complaining of. You might have considered a risk diagnosis for communication and how to ensure that Mabel understood the head injury guidance given. The defining characteristics of these diagnoses, according to Carpenito-Moyet (2013), would be as follows:

- nausea – wave-like sensation with salivation, pallor and tachycardia, subjective descriptions;
- confusion – disorientation, fear and anxiety;
- pain – the patient reports and describes the sensation and intensity of painful stimuli;
- congruence between verbal and non-verbal message.

Further reading

Carpenito-Moyet, LJ (2013) *Handbook of Nursing Diagnosis*, 14th edn. Philadelphia: Wolters Kluwer Health/Lippincott Williams Wilkins.

This book identifies the history of nursing diagnosis and some of the issues nurses have with the concept and sets out in detail the features and characteristics of a variety of nursing diagnoses. It is especially useful for the novice practitioner.

Useful website

www.nanda.org
This website contains the NANDA nursing diagnoses guidelines and updated information.

Chapter 6
Care-planning principles
Lioba Howatson-Jones

> **NMC Standards for Pre-registration Nursing Education**
>
> This chapter will address the following competencies:
>
> **Domain 3: Nursing practice and decision-making**
> 4. All nurses must ascertain and respond to the physical, social and psychological needs of people, groups and communities. They must then plan, deliver and evaluate safe, competent, person-centred care in partnership with them, paying special attention to changing health needs during different life stages, including progressive illness and death, loss and bereavement.
> 10. All nurses must evaluate their care to improve clinical decision-making, quality and outcomes, using a range of methods, amending the plan of care, where necessary, and communicating changes to others.
>
> **Domain 4: Leadership, management and team working**
> 2. All nurses must systematically evaluate care and ensure that they and others use the findings to help improve people's experience and care outcomes and to shape future services.

> **NMC Essential Skills Clusters**
>
> This chapter will address the following ESCs:
>
> **Cluster: Care, compassion and communication**
> 2. People can trust the newly registered graduate nurse to engage in person-centred care empowering people to make choices about how their needs are met when they are unable to meet them for themselves.
>
> **Cluster: Organisational aspects of care**
> 9. People can trust the newly registered graduate nurse to treat them as partners and work with them to make a holistic and systematic assessment of their needs; to develop a personalised plan that is based on mutual understanding and respect for their individual situation promoting health and well-being, minimising risk of harm and promoting their safety at all times.

Care-planning principles

continued ...

By the second progression point:
10. With the person and under supervision, plans safe and effective care by recording and sharing information based on the assessment.
10. People can trust the newly registered graduate nurse to deliver nursing interventions and evaluate their effectiveness against the agreed assessment and care plan.

By the second progression point:
1. Acts collaboratively with people and their carers enabling and empowering them to take a shared and active role in the delivery and evaluation of nursing interventions.

Chapter aims

After reading this chapter you should be able to:

- explain why care plans are needed;
- identify a nursing problem;
- understand the care-planning stages;
- make the connection between nursing as a therapy and nursing care outcomes;
- develop a written care plan.

Introduction

Case study: Grace's loss of confidence

Grace is 78 years old and lives with her friend, Mary, in a semi-detached house. She suffered a fall recently which has knocked her confidence. Grace is normally an outgoing individual having previously attended many activities such as a reading group and helping out at a local crèche, but she is now scared to leave the house. Mary has severe arthritis and has not been able to help Grace much. A person from their local church has helped do some of the shopping and cleaning. Siobhan, a nurse working with the intermediate care team, picks up Grace's referral and assesses Grace's needs and plans her care. The first thing she observes when visiting Grace at home is that there are many loose rugs downstairs and that the stairs leading up to her first floor bedroom are rather steep with only the main banister for support. There is also a step from the kitchen into the dining area. When Siobhan questions Grace about her eyesight, Grace admits that this has become progressively worse because of her diabetes. Siobhan checks Grace's blood sugar reading and the medication she is taking. The blood sugar reading is within normal limits. When Siobhan questions Grace about what led to her fall, Grace breaks down and says she and Mary had had a row about cooking supper and she was not looking where she was going and tripped and fell. She felt unhappy and depressed and this had worsened since the fall as she did not feel safe going out, but missed her other friends.

Siobhan identifies that Grace has safe environment, mobility and psychological issues which need to be factored into a plan of care. Working with Grace, Siobhan is able to develop a plan of care that includes other

Chapter 6

continued ...

> *professionals such as the occupational therapist to ensure that Grace gets the adaptation aids which will make the house safer, the advice which will empower her to manage to self-care and psychological support which will help address her low mood. Because Siobhan works closely with other professionals like the occupational therapists in the intermediate care team, she is able to share her care plan and discuss some of the planned interventions.*
>
> *Grace's house had an extra handrail fitted to the stairs and a wall-mounted grab rail fitted by the kitchen step. Grace and Mary asked their cleaning helper to remove the loose rugs and when Grace shared the reason why, the helper invited other church members to visit Grace on a regular basis. The next time Siobhan met with Grace she appeared more confident and happier.*

This chapter builds on the previous ones by considering the actions that need to be written into care planning in order to complete the nursing process. This is also helpful for other professionals to understand how nursing actions fit with their priorities. The case study above illustrates how teams work together and can involve different professionals in planning interventions for their patients. It also highlights how the principles of communication, care and commitment – three of the 6Cs – are enacted. This chapter will explain why care plans are needed and how to determine nursing interventions. Through the activities you will be given the opportunity to make the connection between nursing as a therapy and nursing care outcomes and to develop a written care plan.

Why care plans are needed

Care planning is necessary because patients' needs are greater than just their medical needs and therefore will involve different professionals. Creating a personalised care plan can offer benefits for patients, health and social care professionals and the organisations within which they work. Some of these benefits include:

- personalised care – involving patients in deciding what their needs are;
- promoting health – exploring patients' understanding of their problem and providing information as needed to help people achieve a higher level of wellness;
- reducing health inequalities – standardising care helps organisations to share and disseminate good practice;
- stimulating choice – the choices patients make can inform commissioning decisions;
- reducing inefficiency – resources are deployed and used according to needs (DH, 2009).

Consider the case study about Lenny to see how these benefits might be achieved in practice and then answer the questions in Activity 6.1.

> ### Case study: Lenny's long-term mental health condition
>
> *Lenny had started to hide in his room because he was hearing voices and thought his girlfriend Mandy was trying to kill him. Mandy became scared of Lenny and asked their GP Paul for help. Paul came to the house and spoke to Lenny through the door of his room. He could see that Lenny was in need of help, but could*

One way in which you can identify the nursing problem is to use the think-aloud reasoning process which might involve the patient, as appropriate, as well as other professionals (Funkesson et al., 2007). This process identifies the nursing knowledge you are using to explain how the problem has been formulated whilst at the same time also taking note of the patient experience and contribution. When you are aligning nursing problems with patient problems you are working in a person-centred way so that the care-planning process is also person-centred. Person-centred understanding here is based on McCormack and McCance's (2010) way of looking at problems from the person's perspective and empowering the patient to make autonomous decisions (see 'Further reading' at the end of this chapter). Reading the case study on David's anxiety about having a vaccination will help you to understand how to identify nursing problems in a person-centred way.

Case study: David's anxiety about having a vaccination

David is 15 years old and at secondary school. He is due to have his BCG injection (a vaccination against tuberculosis) and all the teenagers in his year queue in the school hall where they are seen by the school nurse, Fiona, for the injection. David is unwilling to have the injection and will not co-operate. He becomes more and more distressed and then walks out, knocking a stack of papers to the floor on his way past.

Fiona decides to talk to David alone later. She meets David in her office the next day and asks him how he is feeling. David tells her that he felt very angry yesterday because he had had a row with his mum at home following the letter sent home from school about the impending injection. David's mum had told him how important it was for him to have this injection and David had told her that he did not understand why he needed it. He found it difficult queuing for the injection and started to feel more and more stressed as he waited with his peers. David described how his heart was racing and he broke out in a cold sweat when approaching the desk where Fiona was giving the injection. He did not want to show himself up in front of his mates and decided it was better to walk out. He did not see the point in having the injection as he did not mix with anyone who was sick and he did not think it was worth the hassle.

Fiona explained to David why the injection was important. She also asked him whether he had ever had any unpleasant experiences with injections. David said that he could remember going to his doctor with his mother as a young child and the nurse talking kindly to him and then putting what felt like a nail in his bottom. He had never forgotten it and whenever he was now approached by health professionals he was very distrustful. Fiona explained that she thought David's anxiety had produced his feeling of panic and psychological unease. Fiona talked David through the injection process, the risks and benefits and offered for David to have the injection in private. She talked through some visualisation techniques with David to help control some of his anxiety. David felt calmer and more in control and asked Fiona to give him the injection now. He practised the techniques that she had taught him while Fiona gave the injection and hardly felt anything. Fiona advised David to talk to his mum about this in case his anxiety recurred in the future.

This case study demonstrates how 'sympathetic presence' is part of a non-judgemental attitude which is essential for building trust and rapport. The case study can also be related to the core value of compassion by taking note of how patients are feeling and being with them. It would have been easy for Fiona to have made a judgement that David was behaving like a typical teenager who did not want to be told what to do. However she realised that there was a problem underlying his behaviour – anxiety – which could be managed as a nursing problem of anxiety due to lack of understanding and fear of pain. By offering some techniques, such as visualisation distraction, where the person thinks of something pleasant and a calm context in which he has previously been happy, Fiona and David managed to work together with the outcome of David having the injection. However Fiona recognises that David's anxiety could recur. By asking him to talk to his mum about it, Fiona is helping David to enlist further support and demonstrating commitment to him through seeking future solutions.

Nursing problems are not always issues that can be dealt with and resolved at the present time. They may require more long-term management going forward. For this reason it is important to recognise that within the care-planning process there will be short- as well as long-term goals. We proceed now to examine the stages of the care-planning process in more detail.

The care-planning stages

You will have already seen that the main stages of the nursing process have been illustrated in Chapter 5 (Figure 5.1, page 71). The stages of care planning follow the nursing process in a similar cyclical way, as follows:

1. identifying the problem and nursing diagnosis – clearly defining what these are from patient assessment information and discussion with the person;
2. establishing the goals – clearly defined benchmarks for measuring achievement of problem-solving which have been agreed with the person;
3. determining nursing interventions – listing nurses' actions based on assessed understanding of the situation and your knowledge and expertise;
4. evaluation of care processes – documenting outcomes of the care given;
5. review dates – the date by which it is expected that a change will have been effected.

The application of the stages is identified in the box below.

As previously mentioned, it is important that you consider both short- and long-term goals and psychosocial as well as physical concerns in order for the care-planning process to be holistic. The stages listed above are easy to recognise within certain fields of nursing, such as within hospital wards; however, they may not be so obvious within the documentation used in ambulatory care areas or the community. Nevertheless, these processes are part of nurses' care-planning thinking, no matter where they work, and therefore it is important to be clear about how this is taking place in order to be able to share the rationale for the decisions you have made about the care of your patient. (You can read more on decision-making in care planning in Chapter 10.) We proceed now to translate some of these principles into developing a written care plan.

Stages of the care-planning process

Stage 1

The patient may have more than one problem, particularly in complex cases. The identified order of the problems will be determined by the nursing model you are using to frame the patient assessment and care-planning process as well as the patient's dependency status. Problems will also be actual as well as potential because the care-planning process includes risk-assessing potential problems. Problems also need to be articulated with reference to nursing. In other words, why are they nursing problems? For example, patient anxiety is a nursing problem because nursing is about making patients feel listened to, comfortable, informed and psychologically safe.

Stage 2

The goal is what the patient will be able to do at the end of a care process, for example, to be able to walk with one stick. Goals need to be formulated in SMART terms. This means that they are specific, measurable, achievable, relevant and time-limited. If goals are too vague it will be difficult to assess progress or to sustain motivation. Goals also need to be short- and long-term, as previously described. Another criterion that can be used when formulating goals is the PRODUCT criteria, described by Barrett et al. (2012) as patient-centred, recordable, observable and measurable, directive, understandable and clear, credible and time-related. There are clear similarities between the SMART and PRODUCT criteria in that they need to be agreed with the patient or service user and clear and measurable within a particular time span. Which one you use will depend on best fit with the patient and context of care.

Stage 3

Determining nursing interventions is about giving specific instructions about what you think nurses need to do in order to address the problem identified and reach the specific goal. Nursing interventions should also be evidence-based and use the latest research (Barrett et al., 2012). They should also incorporate the patient or service user's preferences and individual needs, such as cultural needs. Nursing interventions also need to be realistic and sustainable within the resources available.

Stage 4

When evaluating, it is necessary to revisit the problem definitions and goal statements in order to identify any changes that have occurred and also any modifications that need to be made. Resolution of the problem may not always occur completely and therefore ongoing care may require refining and modifying the definition of the problem and the planned nursing interventions.

Chapter 6

continued ...

Stage 5

The review dates need to be set within a realistic timescale for potential resolution of the particular problem. These are also important for communication between teams and continuity of care. These will ensure that there are particular checkpoints for evaluating a patient's progress and the outcome of care processes. This is also important to make sure that resources are used efficiently and appropriately.

Developing a written care plan

Caring for patients requires a clear vision of what you hope to achieve, who is to carry out the prescribed nursing interventions and how these are progressing (Barrett et al., 2012). An example care plan that includes the stages described above can be found in the box below and Table 6.1.

Example care plan

Tim's assessment

Tim has been admitted to day surgery for a haemorrhoidectomy. Tim is a 50-year-old firefighter. He works shifts which include days and nights. He lives in a semi-detached house with his wife Carol and three children aged 8, 12 and 14 years old. They have no pets. Carol also works shifts as a registered nurse. Tim is a non-smoker and only drinks alcohol on his days off duty. Tim's body mass index is 24. On admission Tim's vital signs are 36.2°C, pulse is 74bpm, respirations are 12 breaths/minute and his blood pressure is 122/82mmHg. Tim will have his operation under general anaesthetic. He is expected to make a sufficient recovery to be able to go home later today after his surgery and be cared for by his wife.

Some common problems with writing care plans are now provided in the following case studies to help you think about how you might avoid them. The associated activities ask you to think critically about the problems and possible solutions.

Case study: Setting goals for Mindi

Mindi has diabetes and a chest infection. The student nurse looking after her has identified a number of problems, one of which is maintaining blood glucose control. She writes the goal as 'able to maintain normal blood glucose levels'.

Activity 6.2   *Critical thinking*

Can you identify any problems with this as a goal when applying SMART principles?

An outline answer is given at the end of the chapter.

Problem	Goal	Nursing interventions	Evaluation	Review date
Anxiety that the operation will have an impact on his ability to work	*Short-term*: Tim's Hospital Anxiety and Depression Scale (HADS) measurement is within the normal range by the time he is discharged from day surgery *Long-term*: Tim is able to work after fourteen days' rest	1. The registered nurse will give Tim time and space to express his anxieties before and after his surgery 2. The registered nurse will provide Tim with information about the procedure and likely effects before the operation and at the point of discharge from day surgery 3. The registered nurse will advise Tim when he is being discharged from day surgery of the precautions to take to avoid complications 4. The registered nurse will check Tim's anxiety using the HADS prior to surgery and prior to discharge and will communicate results to the team	Tim expressed his concerns about getting back to work and being able to do what he did before. The operation procedure has been explained to Tim by the surgeon and the registered nurse and he understands that he will not be able to undertake firefighting duties for 14 days. Tim has been advised of the need to avoid constipation and of the signs of infection. Tim has been given the out-of-hours number for day surgery	Next day
Postoperative pain and nausea	*Short-term*: Tim's pain and nausea will be controlled with postoperative medication *Long-term*: Tim will not have any pain or nausea after 14 days	1. The registered nurse will check Tim's pain and nausea score on return from surgery, after an hour and prior to discharge 2. The registered/assistant nurse will position Tim comfortably 3. The registered nurse will ensure that Tim has pain medication to take home and understands how to take it	Tim's pain score on return from surgery was 3 and his nausea score was 1. He was given prescribed pain and nausea medication by the registered nurse which alleviated his symptoms. By the time he was discharged, Tim's pain and nausea scores were 0. He understood how to take his medication and that he could not drink alcohol or operate machinery whilst taking it. Tim and his wife understood that	On return from theatre

continued...

Problem	Goal	Nursing interventions	Evaluation	Review date
		4. The registered nurse will instruct Tim and his wife where to seek further help if his pain or nausea worsens when he is at home	they needed to speak to their GP if his pain or nausea worsened. Tim's pain lasted 12 days and he was able to go back to light duties after 14 days off sick	
Cognitive ability and orientation to time and place	*Short-term*: Tim will be fully oriented to time and place on discharge *Long-term*: Tim will be able to process decision-making information cognitively after 24 hours	1. The registered/assistant nurse will give Tim time to wake up slowly 2. The registered/assistant nurse will tell Tim that he has returned to the ward and what the time is 3. The registered nurse will check Tim's sedation score 4. The registered nurse will offer explanations when Tim is fully awake	Tim was sleepy on his return to the ward from theatre with a sedation score of 3. He did ask twice what the time was. On discharge Tim was fully oriented to time and place, although he still felt a bit tired and was therefore advised to rest when he got home	On return from theatre
Actual problem: Surgical rectal wound *Potential problem*: Infection	Wound shows signs of healing and absence of infection by end of week 1	1. The registered nurse will observe the wound for any bleeding postoperatively prior to discharge 2. The registered nurse will advise Tim how to care for the wound at home 3. The registered nurse will advise Tim and his wife of the signs of infection and to seek help from his GP if any of these occur	Tim's wound showed some minimal bleeding on the pad. He was able to remove the pad after three days. He followed the instructions regarding avoiding constipation, resting for 14 days and returning to light duties and his wound healed well without incident	Next day
Long-term problem: Further haemorrhoids	Tim is maintaining a high fibre diet by day 7	1. The registered/assistant nurse advise Tim about high fibre diet options 2. The registered nurse will advise drinking at least 2 litres of water per day.	On discharge from day surgery, Tim knew what dietary and fluid options were helpful for his recovery	On discharge

Table 6.1: Example care plan (see also the box on page 86)

> **Case study: Prescribing nursing interventions for George**
>
> *George has had a stroke. He has recovered some of his speech, but remains immobile. He is very depressed and finds it difficult to accept that other people need to carry out his care needs. The student nurse looking after George plans the following nursing interventions.*
>
> - *Give all care to George.*
> - *Refer to a counsellor.*
> - *Refer to the occupational therapist.*
> - *Refer to the physiotherapist.*
> - *Complete an anxiety and depression scale score.*

Activity 6.3 — Critical thinking

Can you identify any problems with these nursing interventions?

An outline answer is given at the end of the chapter.

The following activity will help you to reflect on what you have learned so far about care planning and how you can apply this knowledge in practice.

Activity 6.4 — Reflection

What are the main points that you need to remember when developing a care plan? How should you formulate goals? How can you ensure that your care-planning process is person-centred and includes core values from the 6Cs as appropriate?

On your next placement try to use the principles introduced in this chapter to develop a care plan with your patient and discuss it with your mentor to see whether you have succeeded.

An outline answer is given at the end of the chapter.

The connection between nursing therapy and nursing care outcomes

Nursing seeks to support patients emotionally, psychologically and physically. As a nurse you will need to find ways of being with the patient that enable you to develop a therapeutic relationship and a 'sympathetic presence', which means that patients feel you understand their point of view. But at the same time you also need to work systematically to achieve agreed goals. Nursing is reflected *not in what we do, but in the way we provide care* (Hawkey and Williams, 2007, p8).

Nurses have the greatest contact time with patients and it is in how you use that contact time that nursing becomes therapeutic rather than a task. Nursing care outcomes, therefore, are centred on the person within the patient rather than a medical diagnosis. Nevertheless, the professional background of staff involved with a care setting or patient will influence the approach to care planning and the way that this is implemented (Worden and Challis, 2008). Concept mapping is one way in which it is possible to gain a holistic nursing view of the person rather than one based on a disease process model (Taylor and Wros, 2007). In concept mapping, assessment information is sorted into clusters to identify problem areas and consider relationships between them. This is a dynamic process which considers gaps in knowledge and information and develops understanding of the complexities of patients' situations. In this way, how you develop the therapeutic relationship with the patient can also be related to the nursing outcomes to assess the effectiveness of your care planning and nursing care.

Conclusion

Care planning that is person-centred is based on developing a therapeutic relationship that recognises the person within the patient and concentrates on how care strategies are decided. Care planning in this way will require you to nurture and develop your way of being with the patient. In the busy health and social care environment, taking time with people may be difficult but is also extremely rewarding in terms of achieving nursing outcomes and quality nursing care and developing working with the core values of the 6Cs.

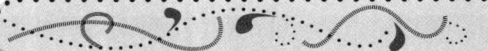

Chapter summary

This chapter has explored why care planning is important for good and effective patient care. It has examined how the process of care planning relates to the nursing process and the different stages involved. You have been given the opportunity to avoid some of the pitfalls in care planning and to develop a care plan of your own. Consideration of how nursing therapy relates to nursing outcomes has promoted reflection on your nursing practice.

Activities: brief outline answers

Activity 6.1 Critical thinking [page 82]

The following questions will help you to identify why care plans are useful in a particular setting.

- What type of care plans are used here?
- How are care plans used?
- Do care plans follow the same format for each patient/condition?
- Are they based on a particular nursing model/philosophy?
- Are patients/carers always involved in the care plan or are there exceptions?
- If so, what are these exceptions?

Health inequalities might be reduced by considering how individual patient needs and planning might translate more widely and give mental health patients optimum chances and access to resources.

Activity 6.2 Critical thinking [page 86]

You might have questioned what is meant by normal, what is the timeframe and how this will be measured when writing an appropriate goal. You might have considered a better goal might be 'will maintain blood sugar levels between 5 and 8mmol over the next seven days, measured by glucometer'. This sets out exactly the conditions to be measured and how this will be done.

Activity 6.3 Critical thinking [page 89]

You might have identified firstly, that these are not nursing interventions because many of them do not involve nurses and secondly, there does not appear to be any involvement of George within these planned interventions. Therefore, nursing interventions might more appropriately include the following.

- Give George the time and space to express how he feels.
- Attentively listen to George to find out what his concerns and priorities are and how he wishes to proceed with the way that he is cared for.
- Offer George some strategies for assisting with his care.

This plan is more person-centred in its approach because it involves George in setting the priorities and in decision-making. While the referrals may be part of the care plan, they should not be the first solution because they are not in themselves nursing interventions.

Activity 6.4 Reflection [page 89]

You might have identified the importance of adopting a person-centred approach to assessment and care planning. This means identifying patient priorities and aligning these with nursing problems. You may have considered the different stages of care planning as: identifying the problem, establishing goals that are specific, measurable, achievable, relevant and time-limited. You might have considered that talking to patients and giving them the time and space to express their needs and discuss care options and strategies was an appropriate way to promote person-centred decision-making and implement working with the core values of the 6Cs.

Further Reading

Barrett, D, Wilson, B and Woollands, A (2012) *Care Planning: A Guide for Nurses*. Harlow: Pearson Education.

This book gives a step-by-step guide to the care-planning process and considers some nursing models which might frame it.

McCormack, B and McCance, T (2010) *Person-Centred Nursing Theory and Practice*. Oxford: Wiley-Blackwell.

This book offers a comprehensive and contemporaneous guide to person-centred nursing practice.

Useful websites

www.mentalhealthcare.org.uk/mental_health_uk

Department of Health run website giving details of the Mental Health Act (1983).

www.ombudsman.org.uk

This website contains a number of case studies about situations where care has been lacking, has not been person-centred or where it has gone wrong. Applying the principles of this chapter to those case studies might help you to understand the importance of care planning for better outcomes.

Chapter 7
Relationship of nursing models to care planning

Lioba Howatson-Jones

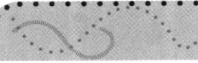

NMC Standards for Pre-registration Nursing Education

This chapter will address the following competencies:

Domain 3: Nursing practice and decision-making
8. All nurses must provide educational support, facilitation skills and therapeutic nursing interventions to optimise health and wellbeing. They must promote self-care and management whenever possible, helping people to make choices about their healthcare needs, involving families and carers where appropriate, to maximise their ability to care for themselves.

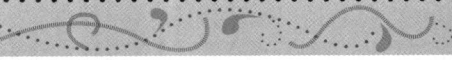

NMC Essential Skills Clusters

This chapter will address the following ESCs:

Cluster: Care, compassion and communication
6. People can trust the newly registered graduate nurse to engage therapeutically and actively listen to their needs and concerns, responding using skills that are helpful, providing information that is clear, accurate, meaningful and free from jargon.

By the first progression point:
1. Communicates effectively both orally and in writing, so that the meaning is always clear.
2. Records information accurately and clearly on the basis of observation and communication.

By the second progression point:
6. Uses strategies to enhance communication and remove barriers to effective communication, minimising risk to people from lack of or poor communication.

Cluster: Organisational aspects of care
9. People can trust the newly registered graduate nurse to treat them as partners and work with them to make a holistic and systematic assessment of their needs; to develop a personalised plan that is based on mutual understanding and respect for their individual situation promoting health and well-being, minimising risk of harm and promoting their safety at all times.

By the second progression point:
10. With the person and under supervision, plans safe and effective care by recording and sharing information based on the assessment.
9. People can trust the newly registered graduate nurse to deliver nursing interventions and evaluate their effectiveness against the agreed assessment and care plan.

Chapter aims

The aim of this chapter is to enable students to understand the relevance of nursing models to the care-planning process. After reading this chapter you should be able to:

- describe a variety of nursing models;
- identify why nursing models are important;
- explain how a nursing model frames the assessment process;
- understand how a nursing model impacts on decision-making in care planning.

Introduction

Case study: Deena's asthma attack

Deena is a 50-year-old accountant who has suffered from asthma ever since she was a child. Her job is pressurised and can be stressful, particularly at certain times of the year when accounts need to be finalised for tax purposes. She takes medication for her asthma and has additional inhalers to use if she has an asthma attack.

It is autumn and the weather has become cold and damp. Deena had her flu vaccination two weeks ago as she was deemed to be at risk. Yesterday, Deena woke up with a wheezy chest and her shortness of breath quite quickly became worse. She used her inhalers, but they did not help. Her husband called an ambulance and Deena was admitted to hospital. Deena was admitted to the respiratory ward by Laura, who is a student nurse. Laura identified that the appropriate nursing model to frame Deena's assessment and care plan was Roper, Logan and Tierney's activities of daily living, because this model helps to consider which areas of Deena's activity are compromised and how these can be improved. The model is also sufficiently systematic to ensure that areas that might at present not be compromised are also considered.

Laura assesses how Deena is currently compromised in the areas of daily living, including: maintaining a safe environment, breathing, communication, controlling body temperature, eating and drinking, washing and dressing, mobilisation, expressing sexuality, death and dying, elimination, working and playing, and sleeping. She identifies that the greatest priorities at the moment are breathing, communication and mobility because Deena is short of breath. Laura's care planning therefore initially focuses on these areas and on nursing interventions which can be employed to help Deena. These include offering reassurance and

Chapter 7

continued ...

> *explaining nursing actions, positioning Deena to aid her breathing, administering and monitoring the effects of prescribed medication and undertaking nursing observations. When Deena's breathing improves the nursing action will be to assist her to mobilise slowly and help her with personal hygiene needs. In terms of eating and drinking, the priority at the moment is to keep Deena hydrated.*
>
> *Deena remained in hospital for a week where she was treated for a chest infection. She was discharged and returned to work after a further two weeks.*

Using a nursing model as a framework helps direct practitioners in their assessment and care-planning process. As the case study above has illustrated, the choice of nursing model directs what is assessed and gives direction for planning nursing interventions, particularly with regard to the focus of those interventions. This chapter will consider a number of nursing models and explore some of the main differences between them and how these relate to care planning. The chapter will also make the link between the nursing model and decisions made in the care-planning process.

Why nursing models are important

There are different specialties of nursing and therefore the nursing approach will also need to be varied. For example, nursing a patient with intensive care needs is different from nursing a patient in an ambulatory care environment, in the community, or in a mental health setting. Equally, patients themselves are unique with their own differing needs. A one-size-fits-all model is therefore neither desirable nor practical, as it does not deal with the complexity of patients' health or personal needs. Nursing models were developed to reflect the nursing values and beliefs associated with nursing and to help articulate the focus and purpose of nursing activity. Nursing models also identify how nursing priorities and concerns can be different from medicine (Barrett et al., 2012). While particular specialties may espouse certain nursing models, these models will always be aligned with the patient's presenting needs and wishes in order to ensure that a holistic assessment and care plan are achieved. Completing Activity 7.1 will help you to think about why nursing models are important for the assessment and care-planning process.

Activity 7.1 — Reflection

Think about the nursing models you have seen used in practice. Consider the following questions.

- How did the model reflect the values and beliefs of the practice area?
- What was the impact of the model on the assessment and care-planning process?
- If there was no nursing model in evidence, how were you able to justify what you were doing?
- How can you integrate working with the 6Cs?

Although this activity is based on your experience, there is a limited outline answer at the end of the chapter.

Relationship of nursing models to care planning

It may sometimes appear that no nursing model is being used in a practice area because care pathway documentation is used instead. Care pathways (sometimes known as integrated care pathways) are multidisciplinary because different professional groups can use them to record their activity with a patient and document their instructions and plans. Care pathways apply to a particular group of patients with similar problems. They often list specific criteria and actions (Barrett et al., 2012). Nevertheless, the framing of patient problems and evaluation of care will usually be based on the values and beliefs stemming from a particular nursing model. Therefore, what can on the surface appear to be working to a medical model by focusing on rectifying health deficits will often also be defined and underpinned by nursing principles based on the expertise of the practitioner. The recent emergence of interest in the 6Cs means that these need to be considered in terms of how they are integrated into the use of the nursing model in ways that are meaningful for different people. It is important to be clear how you describe and justify your nursing activity in order to communicate this accurately to the patient or service user, as well as to other members of the nursing and interprofessional team.

Nursing models

Nursing models are based on the environment of care, the people involved in nursing activity, the health status of the patient or service user and nursing capabilities and knowledge of the practitioner (Hinchliff et al., 2008). The nursing model explains how we will complete the different stages of the nursing process (Aggleton and Chalmers, 2000) (for more information on the nursing process, revisit Chapter 5). In addition, nursing models help to identify the appropriate assessment tools to use to help with the problem-solving process (for more on assessment tools, revisit Chapter 4). Linking the nursing model with the nursing process will enable you to deliver consistent and evidence-based nursing care where you critically examine the basis of your problem-solving and accurately and contemporaneously document the process (Dyson, 2004). Remember that, in legal terms, if it is not documented it did not happen. Completing Activity 7.2 will help you to identify some of the skills required of the practitioner for using a nursing model.

Activity 7.2 — Critical thinking

What skills, including the 6Cs, do you think are required of the practitioner when using a nursing model?

An outline answer is given at the end of the chapter.

You might have thought about communication and assessment skills, but the skills required of the practitioner are more far-ranging than these. There are many nursing models available as nursing theorists think about how nursing activity can be appropriately articulated and framed. The nursing models in use are also being adapted and updated because of the dynamic nature of healthcare and the diversity of service users. We will look at four of the main nursing models in use in this chapter. These are:

1. Roy's adaptation model;
2. Roper–Logan–Tierney's activities of daily living;
3. Orem's self-care model;
4. Neuman's system.

Each model will be followed by a case study to demonstrate application of the model to patient care.

Roy's adaptation model (Hinchliff et al., 2008)

The aim of this model is to help the patient to develop coping strategies for different health statuses. These are:

- physiological;
- self-concept;
- role functions;
- interdependence.

The assessment focuses on stimuli and stressors that underpin these in terms of the main cause of the problem, factors which can influence the problem and the beliefs and attitudes of the patient about the situation. Now read the following case study to see how the principles might be applied.

Case study: Enid's adjustment to the beginning of dementia

Enid was in her mid-70s. She lived with her granddaughter, Imogen, and was very close to the family. Recently she had started to forget things and was often found wandering in the street. Imogen took her to see the doctor. Enid was referred and seen by a consultant who diagnosed the beginning of dementia. Enid was devastated by this news, as was Imogen. The nurse, Ivy, talked through the diagnosis with Enid and Imogen. Because the diagnosis of dementia meant a lot of adjustments for Enid and Imogen, Ivy decided to use Roy's adaptation model to frame her assessment and care planning with Enid. Ivy asked Enid and Imogen to describe their daily life in order to identify potential triggers for Enid's change in behaviour. Ivy's assessment focused on:

- *how Enid thought about herself;*
- *Enid's relationship with her granddaughter;*
- *Enid's role in the family;*
- *any physical effects Enid was experiencing.*

Ivy created a plan of care with Enid and Imogen which took into account their wishes and lifestyle. Ivy began by discussing their understanding of dementia. A short-term goal that Ivy identified was to increase their knowledge of dementia in order to give them confidence in how to deal with it. Goal achievement would be evidenced if Enid and Imogen felt less anxious by the time they left the clinic. A longer-term goal was that

> *Enid's relationship with her granddaughter was strengthened as her dependency increased. Therefore Ivy recommended that Enid and Imogen talked about their shared history regularly and used photos to revisit significant events. Goal achievement would be evidenced by Enid being able to remember and engage with Imogen by talking about some past events. Ivy also suggested that Imogen tried to involve Enid in family activities. The goal here was to maintain and support Enid's role in the family for as long as possible.*

In the case study above you will have noted that Ivy's assessment of Enid has identified anxiety stemming from the medical diagnosis of early dementia. She has planned care that includes providing information about early dementia and ways of coping with it. It is important to recognise that, even in short-term care environments such as an outpatient clinic, nurses still use nursing models to underpin their assessment and care planning with the patient. Completing Activity 7.3 will help you to identify other possible aspects that have not been mentioned in the case study.

Activity 7.3 — *Critical thinking*

Read the case study about Enid again and consider the following questions.

- What other aspects of Enid's self-concept might you consider?
- What other aspects of Enid's relationship with her granddaughter might you want to think about?
- What physical aspects might also need to be considered?
- How is Ivy demonstrating using the 6Cs?

An outline answer is given at the end of the chapter.

We proceed now to explore the use of Roper, Logan and Tierney's activities of daily living model.

Roper, Logan and Tierney's activities of daily living (Roper et al., 2000)

The aim of this model is to consider factors which comprise daily living, in a holistic and systematic way. The model takes account of 12 arenas that make up daily living:

1. maintaining a safe environment;
2. communicating;
3. breathing;
4. eating and drinking;
5. controlling body temperature;
6. washing and dressing;
7. working and playing;

8. mobilising;
9. eliminating;
10. expressing sexuality;
11. sleeping;
12. dying.

The assessment focuses on all the areas and plans nursing interventions within those areas that are compromised, or potentially compromised. Now read the following case study to see how the principles might be applied.

> ### Case study: Murdo's trip to the seaside
>
> *You are on a learning disability placement and this week the residents have a trip organised to go to the seaside. You are going with them and are responsible for Murdo. Murdo is a 14-year-old boy who has Down's syndrome. You check his care plan in order to identify what care you should be giving him. The care plan identifies that Murdo requires some help with washing and dressing and that he occasionally becomes frustrated, leading to angry outbursts when in unfamiliar situations. He likes helping in the garden and enjoys art. You note that Murdo does not appear to have any problems with eating and drinking or elimination. He is quite affectionate with people, which can sometimes be taken the wrong way.*
>
> *You talk with Murdo before the trip to find out how he feels about it and what he wants to do. Murdo says that he wants to find some shells so that he can make a picture. He also wants to paddle in the sea. You ask Murdo what he thinks the seaside will be like and who will be there. Murdo says that he thinks there will be sand and water and shells. You tell Murdo that there will be a lot of people there whom he will not know, and that it might be a good idea if he walks with you. You also suggest that he should tell you if he does not like something. You plan to bring drawing materials with you so that Murdo can draw a picture of the seaside. You plan to use drawing as a distraction if Murdo becomes agitated and frustrated, to try and avoid an outburst.*
>
> *The trip to the seaside goes well. Murdo did want to give the waitress in the cafe a hug and you were able to explain that he was showing appreciation for the meal and the service. Murdo did become frustrated when told that he had to leave the seaside. You suggested that he started to think about a picture of his day at the seaside on the way back to the bus and then gave him the drawing materials on the bus to complete the picture.*

In the case study above you will have noted the communication used to prepare Murdo for his trip to the seaside. You will also have seen how a safe environment is maintained through suitable distraction techniques and supervision. Murdo's expression of his sexuality in his affectionate approach to others is appropriately explained so that there is no offence taken.

It is important to recognise that this model is suitable for use across a range of nursing contexts and settings. Completing Activity 7.4 will help you to consider the application of some of the other activities of daily living.

Relationship of nursing models to care planning

Activity 7.4 — Critical thinking

Read the above case study again and consider the following questions.

- What other activities of daily living might be relevant here?
- What other aspects of maintaining a safe environment might need to be considered?
- In what way are the principles of the 6Cs demonstrated here?

An outline answer is given at the end of the chapter.

We proceed now to explore the use of Orem's (2001) self-care model.

Orem's self-care model (Orem, 2001)

This model recognises that people have capabilities and limitations for self-care as follows:

- self-care agency – relates to being able to take deliberate action to achieve desired goals, e.g. getting out of bed;
- universal self-care requisites – relates to what we need to take in in order to stay alive, e.g. fluid, food, air;
- developmental self-care requisites – relates to physical, functional and psychological development across the lifespan;
- health deviation self-care requisites – means how disorders can interfere with acquiring what is needed;
- helping methods and nursing systems – actions taken to help compensate or overcome limitations to patients' ability to act;
- self-care deficit – something that individuals might do for themselves but for which they require help due to limitations in capabilities, such as cognitive, physical or psychological ability. Deficits might be needing support with washing, moving about or decision-making, for example.

Nursing action is required to support individuals in dealing with limitations to their ability to be self-caring. The therapeutic relationship we build with patients influences the assessment of their response to whether they are managing or whether they need our help and support. Now read the following case study to see how the principles might be applied.

Case study: Patrick's rugby accident

Patrick had been playing rugby last Saturday and sustained a shoulder injury which required surgery. His shoulder has been strapped following the surgery and he will be out of action for three months. Patrick is normally fit and well and is in his late 20s. He will only need to stay in hospital for a couple of days. However, due to his shoulder being strapped he requires some help with washing and dressing and will not be able to carry things when he gets home. Sleeping is also awkward because he finds lying in bed painful.

> *Patrick is getting fed up with being reliant on other people to help him. His nurse Aisling identifies that he has self-care deficits in that he will require nursing intervention to assist him with washing and dressing. He will also require pain relief and help with positioning at night to assist him to sleep. Aisling shows him ways in which he can help himself with getting dressed. She also discusses with Patrick and his wife Niamh how to continue when he is at home. By identifying what he can still do, Aisling has helped ease some of Patrick's frustration and he goes home in a better frame of mind to support his recovery and return to self-care.*

In the above case study about Patrick you may have noticed some of the helping roles which the nurse took in accordance with Orem's (2001) model. These include:

- partly compensatory, as the nurse assists with his washing and dressing but allows Patrick a role as well by guiding him to what he can do;
- wholly compensatory, by making sure he does not lift anything;
- teaching him about the best position for sleeping and how to take his medication;
- supporting him by offering psychological support to deal with his frustration.

Completing Activity 7.5 will help you to consider other capabilities and limitations for self-care.

Activity 7.5 — Critical thinking

Read the above case study again and consider the following questions.

- What other nursing systems could Aisling use to help in her care planning for Patrick?
- What other limitations on self-care might also need to be considered?

An outline answer is given at the end of the chapter.

We proceed now to explore Neuman's system.

Neuman's system (Barrett et al., 2012)

This system is based on features that make us who we are, but which can also be variables that interact with each other in different ways depending on stress and personal factors. These are:

- physiological – relating to the anatomy and physiology of the person;
- psychological – relating to mental states, relationships and interaction with other people;
- sociocultural – with regard to background, beliefs and norms;
- developmental – relating to physical and psychological lifespan changes;
- spiritual – with regard to belief systems.

Neuman sees health as a continuum of wellbeing which is constantly adapting to the environment (Barrett et al., 2012). Stressors arise from the internal and external environment and individual lines of resistance used to try and mediate these threats. Now read the following case study to see how the principles might be applied.

> ### Case study: Andrea's new baby
>
> *Andrea is 29 years old and has come into hospital to have her first baby. Her job is a nursing sister in a care home. Her husband has recently been made redundant and her family live mostly abroad. She has a sister who lives 200 miles away. She started her maternity leave a month ago and was planning to take three months off work. However her husband's redundancy means that she will have to go back to work as soon as possible.*
>
> *Following the birth of her daughter Andrea appears withdrawn and does not seem to be sleeping very well. The baby is well cared for and Andrea responds to her baby's needs appropriately. Mimi, the midwife caring for Andrea, is concerned for her wellbeing. She wonders whether the stresses which Andrea has experienced with her husband losing his job and now the new baby bringing changes to their relationship will overwhelm Andrea's lines of resistance, which include her professional knowledge of healthcare and some family support (albeit at a distance). Mimi decides to speak to Andrea about her situation and offer some advice and guidance. She will also check Andrea for postnatal depression and get her seen by a doctor as well.*
>
> *It is clear from Mimi's assessment of Andrea that she is developing depression. Mimi talks to Andrea and her husband John about what they can do to minimise the effects and build up Andrea's defences. She shows them some relaxation techniques. The doctor also prescribes medication to help Andrea.*
>
> *Andrea goes home at the end of the week when her baby has regained her birth weight. Her sister comes to stay to help her out, and the community midwife and health visitor both check on the progress of both Andrea and her daughter. With this support in place, Andrea seems to be more able to cope. She continues on the medication for another month, and seems more communicative and engaged with the people around her.*

Completing Activity 7.6 will help you to consider other stressors and lines of resistance which may also be relevant when using this model.

Activity 7.6 — Critical thinking

Read the above case study again and consider the following questions.

- What other stressors might Andrea have?
- What other lines of resistance are available to her?
- What else could Mimi do?
- Which of the 6Cs is Mimi using here?

An outline answer is given at the end of the chapter.

We proceed now to looking at how a nursing model frames the assessment process.

Chapter 7

How a nursing model frames the assessment process

Aggleton and Chalmers (2000, p11) state that:

> *The use of an appropriate nursing model informs assessment by establishing the kind of information required, the detail that is likely to be helpful and the ways in which the information might be best gathered.*

The nursing model provides the conceptual framework from which activity flows. Dougherty and Lister (2008, p29) further identify that:

> *Structuring patient assessment is vital to monitor the success of care and to detect the emergence of new problems. Nursing models provide frameworks for a systematic approach to assessment.*

What this means is that if you are using a nursing model to frame the assessment process, it will ensure that you focus on relevant areas and are less likely to miss important cues. Table 7.1 sets out the different foci for assessment of the nursing models identified above.

Now read the following case study and complete Activity 7.7 in order to apply the different approaches to assessment relating to the different nursing models.

> ### Case study: Bradley's development of epilepsy
>
> *Bradley is a mechanic. He is in his early 20s. After a night out with his mates 6 months ago he was taken to hospital following a seizure. A number of tests were completed which showed that he had epilepsy. Bradley has found it difficult to come to terms with this diagnosis. He had to change his job because of not being able to drive and now works for the council in the parks and gardens. The money is less which is a worry for him. Three months ago Bradley met a girl and they are becoming quite serious about each other. She is learning to cope with his fits. However, after another night out with his friends he again is brought to accident and emergency with a longer seizure.*

Activity 7.7   *Critical thinking*

Using the case study and Table 7.1, identify the main assessment points for Bradley when using the selected nursing models.

An outline answer is given at the end of the chapter.

Nursing model	Focus of assessment
Roy's adaptation model (Aggleton and Chalmers, 2000)	Adaptive problems, for example, learning to live with a long-term condition. Patient experience, for example, their narrative and description of how this is for them. Nursing diagnosis, for example, anxiety about the developing relationship, not losing his girlfriend or job.
Roper–Logan–Tierney activities of daily living (Roper et al., 2000)	Biographical and health information such as the person's name, age, personal circumstances and reason for seeking health professional input. The person's ability to carry out the activities of daily living. Risk-assessing potential problems, for example, personal injury during a fit.
Orem's self-care model (Orem, 2001)	Self-care capabilities – what resources and knowledge does the person have to be self-caring? What are the person's routines? Self-care limitations – what interferes with a person being able to self-care? Self-care agency – how has the person managed problems with being able to self-care?
Neuman's system (Barrett et al., 2009)	Person's perception of their situation, for example what are their health concerns? The effect of stressors on the person, for example, how are things different? Your perception of the person and their situation, for example what do you see as the person's problem and why?

Table 7.1: Foci for assessment with different nursing models

We now proceed to look at how nursing models also have an impact on decision-making in care planning (see also Chapter 10 on decision-making in care planning).

How a nursing model impacts on decision-making in care planning

As identified above, a nursing model directs the focus of assessment and through this process also influences the decisions made for planning care. The transition from assessment to care planning involves critical thinking and clinical reasoning (Aston et al., 2010). Critical thinking means:

- evaluating assessment information;
- forming judgements about the information you have.

When you are at the start of your preparation programme you will probably follow the nursing model cues unquestioningly. However, as you develop knowledge and skill, you will start reasoning how applicable the model is for the patient's needs and consider the appropriate evidence to use for your care planning. Table 7.2 sets out the main considerations for decision-making in care planning for the nursing models identified above.

Nursing model	Focus of care planning
Roy's adaptation model (Aggleton and Chalmers, 2000)	The nursing diagnosis guides the care plan. Goals need to be short- and long-term. Nursing interventions are related to the stimulus for adaptation. Care planning should be evidence-based.
Roper–Logan–Tierney activities of daily living (Roper et al., 2000)	Helping people to return to independence. Teaching people what they need to know. Communicating information.
Orem's self-care model (Orem, 2001)	Prescribing nursing operations, which means the nursing interventions needed. Supporting self-care agency, which means involving individuals in their own care planning.
Neuman's system (Barrett et al., 2009)	Prioritising goals. Prevention as intervention, which means preventing someone either becoming unwell or becoming worse if already unwell.

Table 7.2: Care planning

Activity 7.8 — Decision-making

Read Bradley's case study again and now apply the different approaches to care planning when using the selected nursing models, as identified in Table 7.2.

An outline answer is given at the end of the chapter.

Conclusion

What has been highlighted is that the approaches stemming from the different nursing models focus on particular aspects of assessment and care decision-making. It is important that you are knowledgeable about a range of nursing models so that you can select the most appropriate for your patient. Systematic assessment and care planning will ensure that you include and integrate all the relevant information from which to formulate the holistic care plan.

Relationship of nursing models to care planning

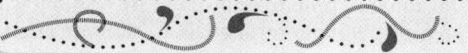

Chapter summary

This chapter has identified the importance of using a range of nursing models to reflect different approaches to care in a variety of settings. These models are important for articulating nursing activity and the values and beliefs that underpin nursing. Summarising application of some of the principles associated with selected nursing models through the case studies supplied and the following activities has given you the opportunity to think critically about how you might use nursing models in practice.

Activities: brief outline answers

Activity 7.1 Reflection [page 94]

You might have identified Roper, Logan and Tierney, Orem, Roy's adaptation model and Neuman's system as nursing models you have seen used in placements. You may have identified that a particular nursing model reflected the level of support required by the patient or service user group in that area. You might also have considered how the model changed the focus of your assessment questioning in terms of whether the patient or service user was returning to self-caring or adapting to a different health status. If there was no nursing model in evidence you might have found yourself having to describe your assessment and care planning 'blind' and therefore potentially from a task-based perspective rather than underpinned by sound nursing principles.

Activity 7.2 Critical thinking [page 95]

The skills required of the practitioner are:

- observation skills;
- communication skills;
- decision-making skills;
- assessment skills;
- nursing diagnostic skills for making a nursing diagnosis;
- critical thinking skills.

The 6C which is used is communication.

Activity 7.3 Critical thinking [page 97]

Other aspects of Enid's self-concept that you might have considered are:

- not knowing who she is any more;
- lack of confidence in herself;
- viewing herself as less capable.

Other aspects of Enid's changing relationship with her granddaughter Imogen which you might have considered are:

- switching of roles as Enid's dependency increases;
- more stressors for the relationship;
- the illness overtaking Enid's identity as a grandmother.

Physical aspects that might need to be considered include:

- deterioration in Enid's short-term memory, which might create safety concerns such as forgetting to turn the oven off, or checking the temperature of food or drink before ingesting, or water before bathing.

Ivy is demonstrating using compassion by allowing Enid and Imogen time to adjust and by working with what is familiar to them. Commitment is demonstrated by looking at longer term goals. Communication is used through the different strategies offered.

Activity 7.4 Critical thinking [page 99]

Other activities of daily living which you might have considered are:

- washing and dressing if Murdo spilt something on himself or was sick;
- elimination in terms of how this would be supervised in a public space.

Other aspects of maintaining a safe environment include what you would do if Murdo did have an angry outburst and how you would manage this. You would need to consider:

- Murdo's safety, making sure that he could not harm himself;
- the safety of others, making sure that they were able to remove themselves from potential harm; your safety.

The 6Cs are demonstrated through the communication used, the care strategies considered and used, and the courage shown in arranging the trip.

Activity 7.5 Critical thinking [page 100]

Other nursing systems that Aisling might have considered include:

- taking a nursing history about patterns of living;
- using pain assessment tools.

As regards limitations on self-care, Patrick may not be able to cut up food and may also require advice with sexual needs.

Activity 7.6 Critical thinking [page 101]

Other stressors for Andrea might be:

- not wanting people to know that she has professional knowledge because it does not relate to children;
- worrying that people expect her to know what to do;
- trying to manage her relationship with her husband at the same time as developing a relationship with her child;
- money worries;
- returning to work so soon.

Other lines of resistance which Andrea could draw on:

- her professional knowledge of caring for others;
- a shared history with her husband;
- continuing more frequent contact with her sister;
- drawing on the experience of work colleagues;
- talking to the mortgage lender and seeking financial advice.

Other areas that Mimi could also consider include:

- referring Andrea to a counsellor and to self-help groups.

Mimi is using the 6Cs through showing her commitment and compassion for Andrea by recognising how she is feeling and working with her and her husband to identify the resources she has. She is also showing her competence in being able to identify these with Andrea.

Activity 7.7 Critical thinking [page 102]

When using Roy's nursing model your assessment is likely to have focused on Bradley's ability to adjust to having epilepsy and still remaining within his circle of friends. Your nursing diagnosis might have been around anxiety relating to knowledge of the condition, and interpersonal and economic factors.

When using Roper, Logan and Tierney's activities of daily living model your assessment is likely to have focused on maintaining a safe environment by assessing Bradley's vital signs and consciousness and considering his ability to carry on working safely. You might also have risk-assessed the potential for Bradley to injure himself while having a fit, and for him to develop depression because of not yet having come to terms with his condition.

When using Orem's nursing model your assessment is likely to have focused on Bradley's ability to take care of himself physically given his lifestyle and the unpredictability of the seizures. You might have identified that he requires nursing support in providing information for him and his girlfriend on ways they can take control of his care.

When using Neuman's system your assessment is likely to have focused on whether Bradley feels stressed and what his main stressor is – is it that he worries about losing this job, or his girlfriend leaving? You would think about discussing this with Bradley to find out how he is feeling and what his perception is. You would also ask how he normally manages his epilepsy and how he wants to be involved in his care. Your perception of Bradley's problem is likely to be that he is a young man in denial of his condition and in a serious relationship which is important to him.

Activity 7.8 Decision-making [page 104]

When using Roy's nursing model your care planning is likely to focus on the nursing diagnosis that Bradley lacks insight into his condition and that he is anxious. The short-term goal which you may consider for Bradley is that he will be fully informed about his condition and treatment within one week. The longer-term goal which you may have identified is that Bradley is less anxious by the end of one week. Your care plan may include stress alleviation strategies such as talking, relaxation techniques and identifying where to get further support, e.g. financial benefits.

When using Roper, Logan and Tierney's model your care plan is likely to focus on communicating information about Bradley's condition and treatment and interpreting this, as appropriate. You might also have considered the nursing observations required, such as neurological observations and positioning Bradley to ensure his breathing is supported. It is likely that you will have also considered teaching Bradley about his medication regimen.

When using Orem's model your care plan is likely to focus on prescribing the nursing interventions required, including educative components, compensatory strategies and support. These are likely to have included informing Bradley about why his seizures follow his nights out and what he can do about this. It is likely that you will involve Bradley in his washing and dressing and talk to him about ways of reducing his anxiety and stress.

When using Neuman's system your care planning is likely to focus on prioritising Bradley's recovery from the seizure and ensuring medication is given on time. You would then consider how to reduce his anxiety and stress to prevent more seizures. You would also need to plan how to help him gain some control through providing information.

Further reading

Aston, L, Wakefield, J and McGown, R (eds) (2010) *The Student Nurse Guide to Decision Making in Practice.* Maidenhead: Open University Press.

This book is useful for outlining the decision-making skills required of the developing nurse and how to make use of evidence and team members to determine a course of action.

Hall, C and Ritchie, D (2012) *What is Nursing?* 3rd edn. London: SAGE/Learning Matters.

An introduction to the world of nursing, incorporating views from student and qualified nurses.

Hinchliff, S, Norman, S and Schober, J (eds) (2008) *Nursing Practice and Health Care*, 5th edn. London: Hodder Arnold.

This book identifies some of the different nursing models, giving examples of their use.

Chapter 8
Ethical aspects of patient assessment dilemmas

Lioba Howatson-Jones

> 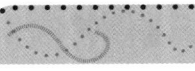   **NMC Standards for Pre-registration Nursing Education**
>
> This chapter will address the following competencies:
>
> **Domain 1: Professional values**
> 1. All nurses must practise with confidence according to *The Code: Standards of conduct, performance and ethics for nurses and midwives* (Nursing and Midwifery Council, 2008), and within other recognised ethical and legal frameworks. They must be able to recognise and address ethical challenges relating to people's choices and decision-making about their care, and act within the law to help them and their families and carers find acceptable solutions.
>
> **Domain 2: Communication and interpersonal skills**
> 8. All nurses must respect individual rights to confidentiality and keep information secure and confidential in accordance with the law and relevant ethical and regulatory frameworks, taking account of local protocols. They must also actively share personal information with others when the interests of safety and protection override the need for confidentiality.

> 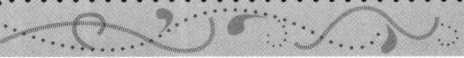   **NMC Essential Skills Clusters**
>
> This chapter will address the following ESCs:
>
> **Cluster: Care, compassion and communication**
> 1. As partners in the care process, people can trust a newly registered graduate nurse to provide collaborative care based on the highest standards, knowledge and competence.
>
> *By the first progression point:*
> 1. Articulates the underpinning values of *The Code: Standards of conduct, performance and ethics for nurses and midwives* (the code) (Nursing and Midwifery Council, 2008).
> 3. People can trust the newly registered graduate nurse to respect them as individuals and strive to help them preserve their dignity at all times.

By the first progression point:
2. Engages with people in a way that ensures dignity is maintained through making appropriate use of the environment, self and skills and adopting an appropriate attitude.
8. People can trust the newly registered graduate nurse to gain their consent based on sound understanding and informed choice prior to any intervention and that their rights in decision-making and consent will be respected and upheld.

By the first progression point:
1. Seeks consent prior to sharing confidential information outside of the professional care team, subject to agreed safeguarding and protection procedures.

By the second progression point:
2. Applies principles of consent in relation to restrictions relating to specific client groups and seeks consent for care.

Cluster: Organisational aspects of care
11. People can trust the newly registered graduate nurse to safeguard children and adults from vulnerable situations and support and protect them from harm.

By the first progression point:
1. Acts within legal frameworks and local policies in relation to safeguarding adults and children who are in vulnerable situations.

Chapter aims

The aim of this chapter is to enable you to develop understanding and application of ethical principles within patient assessment processes. After reading this chapter you will be able to:

- understand the relevance of ethical theories to patient assessment and care planning;
- relate ethical principles such as autonomy, beneficence, non-maleficence and justice to patient assessment;
- identify some problems with ethics as theory and ethics in practice;
- begin to problem-solve ethical dilemmas in patient assessment and resource allocation.

Introduction

Case study: Nancy's ethical dilemma

Nancy is working in a mental health day unit where a number of the older patients who attend have early dementia. One woman, Sybil, has been coming for a number of months and Nancy has built a close

Chapter 8

continued ...

> *therapeutic relationship with her. Sybil lives with her daughter, Marion. Marion works part-time on the days that Sybil is at the day unit. Sybil has recently been complaining to Nancy that her daughter is locking her in her bedroom and hiding her money. She says she has been asking her grandson Luke for money and he has given her some of his pocket money. She says she has been asking Luke to run errands for her such as posting her replies to begging letters. Nancy is concerned about this. She considers whether she can break Sybil's confidentiality and speak to Marion about this as she is concerned about Sybil's vulnerability to scams and the involvement of her grandson.*

Ethics underpin healthcare practice and are written into the code of conduct for nurses and midwives with clear expectations of how practitioners are expected to conduct themselves. The above case study raises ethical issues in relation to confidentiality, autonomy and mental capacity. This chapter will introduce the main ethical theories which encapsulate healthcare practice. It will identify how these relate to patient assessment and care planning. You will be given the opportunity to explore ethical dilemmas relating to patient assessment and care planning after you have had the chance to learn more about ethical principles and will be asked to return to Nancy's case study above to discuss the dilemma described in Activity 8.4. The chapter will also ask you to consider issues about translating ethics as theory into ethics in practice.

Ethical theories

Ethics underpin the justification for the actions that healthcare professionals take (Hendrick, 2000). The two main ethical theories are consequentialism and deontology. We will look at these two theories in a bit more detail now.

Consequentialism considers that the consequences of an action justify how it is carried out. Therefore, if the results benefit the person then this justifies actions taken to reach that goal. This is often justified as the greatest benefit for the most people, which is a utilitarian view. For example, when a new drug becomes available organisations such as the National Institute for Health and Care Excellence will not only consider its efficacy, but also the ethics of distribution in terms of how the greatest number of people can benefit within economic constraints. Read the case study below to help you understand this theory.

> **Case study: Aggi's emergency response**
>
> *Aggi is a registered nurse and was on her way home from work on a bicycle. It was winter and raining. Rounding a corner Aggi found the traffic was at a standstill. Because she was on a bicycle Aggi was able to weave her way through to the front of the queue. She found the cause of the stoppage was an elderly lady lying in the middle of the road having been knocked over by a car. The car driver was standing nearby clearly distressed.*
>
> *Aggi parked her bicycle and started organising things. She first checked that the emergency services had been called and then carried out a swift assessment of the elderly lady. She noted that blood and fluid were oozing*

Ethical aspects of patient assessment dilemmas

from the old lady's ear. Fortunately the old lady was already on her side. Aggi asked for a blanket to keep her warm. She then asked a spectator to sit the distressed driver down and stay with her. She asked another spectator – a man called Charles – to direct the traffic around the injured woman.

The police and ambulance arrived shortly after and Aggi was relieved to hand over.

Activity 8.1 — Critical thinking

How might Aggi's actions be justified if she was called to account for them? What might be the consequences if the elderly lady died?

An outline answer is given at the end of the chapter.

Deontology

Deontology considers the motivation behind actions and whether these are morally just. This is determined by rules and obligations of duty such as are embedded in the code of conduct. The result of this is an expectation of 'doing as you would be done by'. For example, no matter how busy the placement area is, if a patient has been incontinent, they would expect you to help clean them up and not leave them wet. Read the following case study to help you understand this theory.

Case study: Leroy's first shift in accident and emergency

Leroy was on his third placement in an accident and emergency department. A prisoner called Bruce was brought in with a broken arm following an assault in prison. Leroy was asked by his mentor Claire to assist in plastering Bruce's arm.

Claire asked one of the accompanying prison officers, Tony, what had happened to Bruce. Tony replied that Bruce was in prison for rape and therefore a target for other prisoners. They had cornered him during lunch and broken his arm by snapping it across a table.

Leroy was surprised at how calmly Claire took this news and that she spoke kindly to Bruce as she plastered his arm checking he was not in any undue pain. At the end of the procedure Claire explained the plaster observations to Bruce, the prison officers and Leroy. Bruce thanked her and was escorted back to the prison van. Leroy found this all rather difficult to take in.

Activity 8.2 — Reflection

In Chapter 2 you were asked to reflect on situations where you might find it difficult to provide unbiased care. Now put yourself in Leroy's situation and think about how you might react. What do you need to consider in order to give professional and unbiased care?

Although this activity is based on your experience, there is a limited outline answer at the end of the chapter.

The moral theories and principles originally outlined by Hippocrates guide shared ethical thinking in healthcare practice. These are beneficence, non-maleficence, autonomy and justice (Seedhouse, 2009).

Beneficence

Beneficence means doing good for the person. For example, health promotion aims to improve the health of individuals by helping them to help themselves. Such activity would be classed as doing good.

Non-maleficence

Non-maleficence means not doing harm. Risk assessment is a fundamental part of healthcare practices in order to avoid doing harm to patients. It is unlikely that a healthcare practitioner would deliberately set out to do harm to the person in their care (although sadly there have been some exceptions). It is incumbent on healthcare professionals and considered good practice to incorporate risk assessment within the assessment and care-planning process in order to ensure that plans are in place to avoid doing harm (revisit Chapters 6 and 7 to look again at how this can be done).

Autonomy

Autonomy recognises that individuals have the right to make their own decisions. For example, it is up to individuals when they want to get washed or dressed or when they want to go to bed, rather than having to fit in with a health and social care routine. Equally, while it may be considered in patients' interests to stop drinking alcohol or reduce their weight or modify their diet, it is nevertheless their autonomous right to choose whether or not to do so.

Justice

Justice is about the shared benefits and burdens of society. It might also be considered that it is a contract between people whereby if that person has given what is asked, he or she can expect something in return. Health and social care is both a benefit and a burden to society as a whole in terms of receiving and resourcing. For example, consider in vitro fertilisation, where the wish for a child is recognised, but which is limited by rules about eligibility and concerns. Such concerns are about the likelihood of multiple embryos and premature birth with the possibility of disability and burden on society.

We proceed now to consider the relevance of ethical theories for patient assessment and care planning.

The relevance of ethical theories to patient assessment and care planning

Ethical theories inform the philosophies of care which guide health and social care practice and for which practitioners are held accountable by service users (Lloyd, 2010). A philosophy of care is a statement about the values and beliefs which inform practice within a given area and therefore also what can be expected. The moral theories of autonomy, beneficence, non-maleficence and justice have implications for patient assessment and care planning in a number of ways particularly where the principles of the 6Cs have not been observed. The principles of the 6Cs are about demonstrating care and compassion through recognising a person's autonomy and dignity of being. The moral theories are now considered individually.

Autonomy

Autonomy assumes that patients have a right to be involved in shared decisions about their care. Within assessment it is important to gather relevant data without trying to control patients' lifestyle or behaviour because autonomy means that they make their own decisions. Therefore, when planning care, health and social care professionals may make recommendations, but it is up to individuals whether they take these up or not. There are some people who have mental capacity issues. This means that they have difficulty with making some decisions, particularly those which are more complex. The Mental Capacity Act (2005) states that people with mental capacity issues should be supported and involved as much as possible in making their own decisions. When decisions are made on their behalf, those decisions need to be in the person's best interests. Reading the case study about William's deteriorating health may help you to make more sense of this.

Scenario: William's deteriorating health

William is a 72-year-old retired railway worker who lives with his wife in a bungalow. His wife, Marjorie, has noticed that William appears to be becoming more confused. He forgets where he has put things and important dates and she often finds him wandering around the house in the night. William had a fall and sustained a sprained ankle. He is admitted for assessment. Marjorie insists that William cannot do anything for himself and proceeds to tell you that you need to tell him what to do. Marjorie constantly bosses William around. William does appear agitated and confused and says that he wants to go and meet his friends for a pint.

You make Marjorie a cup of tea and ask her to wait outside while you undertake your assessment of William. William is not able to answer a number of your assessment questions and a number of times says that he needs to go. You identify that he has memory problems and therefore is not sure where he is. You tell him where he is on a number of occasions and reinforce this information as required.

You identify that William is capable of expressing a preference for what he likes to eat or drink and whether he wants you to touch his ankle. William is also able to tell you whether he is in pain or not. However you do have concerns about his ability to make decisions about his care arrangements, especially when he is discharged, and you communicate these concerns to the healthcare team.

Activity 8.3 — Critical thinking

The case study above identifies some problems about William being able to make his own decisions. Consider the following questions.

- How is William's autonomy affected?
- What does the Mental Capacity Act (2005) have to say about this? (see 'Useful websites' at the end of this chapter)
- What else might you need to consider?
- How does this relate to the principles of the 6Cs?

An outline answer is given at the end of the chapter.

Beneficence

Beneficence relates to doing good, as identified earlier. With this focus in mind you need to ensure that your assessment considers the welfare of patients and that at all times you are promoting their health. Read the following case study to help you to understand how this might translate into practice.

Case study: Henry's reluctance to engage

Henry is an 81-year-old man who lives with his daughter, Miranda. He has had incontinence issues for some time now and has become more and more reclusive, withdrawing from family interaction and engagement with people in general. The continence nurse has been to visit him and explained options available to help him manage his incontinence. However Henry would rather continue using a bottle, which he misses a lot of the time, thereby soiling his clothing and his bed sheets, which Miranda has to deal with every day. Miranda is at her wits' end and finds Henry's stubbornness very unhelpful.

Henry has a son Graham who lives in the next county. Graham has invited Henry to come and stay so that Miranda gets a break. Henry is concerned about going because of his incontinence problems and refuses to visit Graham. Miranda talks to the community nursing team and asks them if there is anything they can do. The community nurse Jill gets in touch with the continence nurse again and arranges a meeting with Henry. They discuss the urisheath system which will enable Henry to travel without incontinence and might make his life easier when he stays with Graham.

Henry is at first reluctant but as Graham and his wife have a baby daughter, Henry is keen to see his new grandchild and finally agrees to try the new device and go to visit his son. Jill is careful to explain tactfully how to fit the urisheath and how to manage it and allows Henry time to get used to the idea. She leaves the urisheath for Henry to examine in his own time in private. She visits a few times to help Henry become more expert in using it.

Henry visited his son Graham and enjoyed meeting his new granddaughter. He is still continuing to use the urisheath and is now able to engage better with Miranda and her family.

The case study above highlights the need for patient assessment specifically to identify problems and plan solutions which not only have a healthcare benefit but which also promote patient well-being and fit in with patient autonomy. Healthcare recommendations may not always be welcomed immediately but when care planning is shared and the benefits for patients are communicated and clarified in such a way that they can understand, then patients are more likely to see how proposed interventions can help them.

Non-maleficence

Non-maleficence is about not doing harm, as identified earlier. This can also be related to the competence element of the 6Cs. From this perspective the assessment focuses on risk-assessing actual and potential problems. Care planning follows this with nursing interventions to prevent such problems occurring, or to minimise their impact. Read the following case study to help you understand this better in terms of patient assessment and care planning.

Case study: Eve's diabetic foot

Eve is 65 years old and has been a diabetic for the last five years. She has now been prescribed insulin and is finding this very cumbersome because it interrupts her day. Eve normally enjoys going on walking holidays and visiting art galleries, but unfortunately she has started to develop neuropathy as her lack of blood sugar control has damaged the nerve endings in her feet, which makes walking difficult now.

Eleanor is a student nurse on a community placement with the practice nurse. Eve comes to see the practice nurse for her regular check-up. Eleanor notices that the practice nurse Fiona pays special attention to Eve's feet and examines them closely. Eleanor also notices that the skin is discoloured and dry and that Eve's toenails look gnarled and a different colour. Fiona gives Eve advice on how to look after her feet, especially the skin. She refers Eve to the chiropodist for specialist help with her toenails.

When Eve has gone, Eleanor asks Fiona why she did not offer to cut Eve's toenails as they looked rather long. Fiona explains that because Eve is a diabetic there are risks attached to cutting toenails, such as introducing infection through a sharp nail scratching a neighbouring toe, or a nick of the skin. People with diabetes should have chiropody assistance with foot care and that is why she referred Eve to the chiropodist as part of her care. Fiona emphasises that care planning includes risk-assessing potential problems such as infection. Eleanor now appreciates the importance of including potential problems in care-planning processes.

The case study above highlights the importance of risk-assessing potential harm that patients may do themselves as well as any potential harm which may result from health professionals not giving necessary information. Care planning to safeguard the patient may also need to involve other members of the health and social care team.

Justice

Justice within patient assessment and care planning relates to the equitable distribution of nursing interventions, resources and time. Read the following case study to understand how this might relate to practice.

Case study: Elaine's sheet dilemma

It was Christmas on the stroke ward and due to norovirus many staff were off sick and some of the patients were affected too. Consequently the ward was short staffed. Elaine – the nurse in charge – needed to prioritise to ensure the patients received the care they needed. She was on shift with only two other staff – one qualified and one healthcare assistant. Between them they determined who had the priority needs and explained to the patients why they might not be immediately available as they would like. Many of the patients had been incontinent or sick and needed changing. As it was Christmas the ward was short of sheets and none were available from other wards. Elaine made the decision to change all the bottom sheets that were wet and replace these with the top sheet and provide blankets or duvets instead for covering the patients. Those who had also been sick received the last clean sheets available. Although not an ideal solution, nevertheless it meant that all the patients were left clean and comfortable.

The case study above highlights a very real situation where nurses frequently have to problem-solve. Ethical ideas of justice would expect that all the patients with wet beds would be treated equally and receive clean sheets. However, as this case study has demonstrated, equality is not always possible within finite resources and therefore clinical judgement has to play a part. Patient assessment is crucial to this for identifying priorities as well as risk-assessing the potential for harm. This highlights that translating ethics into practice can sometimes be problematic. We proceed now to explore some such problems.

Problems with ethics as theory and ethics in practice

Problems with ethics as theory and ethics in practice often relate to resourcing issues. For example, waiting lists are the result of many people requiring treatment, but limited spaces available or staff to support this. Equally, problems may arise from a mismatch in ethical thinking and ethical behaviour. For example, you may espouse non-discriminatory practice, but may have identified that you do need to discriminate in order to provide necessary care. Aston et al. (2010, p90) make the point that, *In everyday practice there are often situations where it can be difficult to know whether we are truly acting in the patient's best interests.* This is especially true where patients come from different cultures and where you may find it difficult to integrate different world views. Consider the following case study which may help your understanding.

Case study: Biji's sexual assault

Biji is a 20-year-old student studying law at university and is admitted to the gynaecology ward with vaginal injuries after she was raped on the way home from a party. Biji is a Hindu and does not want her family to know because of the shame this would bring on them. She is clearly distressed and in need of support. You

Ethical aspects of patient assessment dilemmas

> *find it hard to understand how this assault could be viewed as her fault by her family. You talk it over with Biji, but she is adamant that she does not want her family to know.*
>
> *Her mother visits that afternoon and asks you what is wrong with Biji. Because Biji has expressly forbidden you telling her family, you say that that information is confidential and she will have to ask Biji herself. Later you see Biji and her mother arguing and when her mother leaves Biji is in floods of tears. You go to comfort her, but she is inconsolable because her mother has disowned her. You try to reassure Biji that her mother will come round, but she says that you do not understand her culture.*
>
> *You are not sure what to do next so you go to speak to your mentor about this. Your mentor identifies that you did the right thing by not breaking Biji's confidentiality and allowing her to make the decision herself about what she told her mother. Nevertheless, it would have been helpful to have had a member of staff there for additional support for Biji when she spoke to her mother. Your mentor advises that you inform yourself about different religious and cultural rules and practices in order to be better prepared in the future.*

Biji's case study highlights how differences in world views can sometimes constrain communication and the therapeutic relationship. Although Biji's confidentiality has not been broken, nevertheless, ethical questions remain about whether this has resulted in doing her good and not doing her harm. Equally the 6Cs highlight that care should also be compassionate, that health professionals should show commitment to patient need and use courage in approaching patients' problems. Moral dilemmas result from the fact that choices need to be made from different alternatives and it may be difficult to predict the consequences of decision-making in practice. For example, a treatment list may need to be cancelled or curtailed and it will be clinicians who decide who is prioritised for treatment. This impinges on the autonomy of individuals to make decisions for themselves. Aston et al. (2010, p91) suggest that we need to consider how good, right, fair, honest and empowering our decision-making is when faced with such ethical dilemmas.

Nurses are morally accountable to do their best for patients (Barrett et al., 2012). In terms of care planning this means accepting responsibility to give good care that is effective, legal and competent. As a student you may feel that you are not always competent to do what is asked of you. It is therefore important that you make known to your mentor, or other team member, that you do not feel proficient to carry out the task and then to follow this up by extending your knowledge. The same applies if a patient asks you to do something that you are not sure about.

Maintaining confidentiality is an area that has been problematic and difficult in ethical terms. Revisit the case study about Nancy's ethical dilemma at the start of the chapter. When you have read the case study again, complete Activity 8.4 in order to problem-solve some of the ethical issues.

Activity 8.4 — Critical thinking

You will have identified some concerns within the case study of Nancy's ethical dilemma. Make a list of what you see as the ethical issues arising in this case. Now answer the following questions.

- What does Nancy need to consider?
- What can Nancy do?
- Who else might Nancy involve?

An outline answer is given at the end of the chapter.

Conclusion

Moral principles in themselves are useful for directing decision-making and actions, but they can also conflict with each other, producing moral and ethical dilemmas. Clinical reasoning can help to problem-solve these dilemmas, but in itself will never be wholly satisfactory or entirely meet a person's needs. It is important for you to recognise this as a part of professional practice and an area for reflection in order to sustain further learning and develop your future practice.

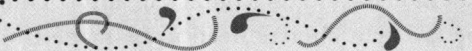

Chapter summary

This chapter has explored the main ethical theories and principles which underpin nursing practice. These have been illustrated through case studies representing some common practice problems. You have been asked to explore critically and reflect on some of the issues raised. In so doing you will have been able to identify some problems with translating ethical theory into ethical practice.

Activities: brief outline answers

Activity 8.1 [page 111]

Aggi is able to justify her actions by showing that she has worked within her limitations and the NMC code of conduct through offering help, making sure the emergency services had been called, completing an assessment and keeping the elderly lady safe from further harm. If the elderly lady subsequently died Aggi would still be able to justify her actions as above. Any arguments would revolve around whether Aggi caused any harm through an action or inaction.

Activity 8.2 [page 111]

It is likely that you would have considered the Nursing and Midwifery Council (2008, 2015) code of conduct, which states that you must not discriminate against people within your care and must treat people kindly and with dignity and respect. You may have identified situations where this might be personally difficult for you. In doing so, it is also important to consider strategies that will help you to overcome these difficulties and to meet and uphold the code of conduct within your practice at all times.

Activity 8.3 [page 114]

William's autonomy is affected by him not knowing where he is and therefore being unable to make informed decisions about whether he stays or goes. In addition, his wife is trying to make decisions for him. The Mental Capacity Act (2005) identifies that, even if he is not able to make complex decisions such as may relate to care arrangements for him when he goes home, nevertheless, he should be consulted on simpler things. For example, what he wishes to eat and drink, whether he wants to wash or get dressed and what he wants to do with his day. It will be important for the healthcare team to determine whether William's decision-making capacity is temporarily or permanently affected. They will also need to consider who can make decisions on his behalf legally, i.e. who has power of attorney? A further consideration that you might have thought about is the relationship between William and his wife Marjorie. Has she an agenda for wanting to take over and make decisions for him? Is this part of their normal relationship? The nurse is demonstrating courage in asking Marjorie to wait elsewhere with a cup of tea. The nurse is using communication to assess what William really perceives of the situation and is demonstrating care in this approach.

Activity 8.4 [page 118]

Your list of what Nancy needs to consider could have included:

- Sybil's autonomy in terms of (allegedly) being locked in her room;
- Sybil's mental capacity;
- the involvement of Sybil's grandson and his collusion;
- Sybil's confidentiality;
- issues of beneficence and non-maleficence, in terms of trying to protect Sybil from being conned and losing all her money, as well as considering the relationship between Sybil and her daughter Marion and grandson Luke.

Nancy firstly needs to speak to Marion to find out some background of what is going on at home. In doing so she is not breaking Sybil's confidentiality. Nancy needs also to consider and assess Sybil's mental capacity and the organisational adult and child protection procedures. If she has concerns within these areas she can then draw on these procedures, particularly as Sybil appears to be a vulnerable adult. Nancy could involve a social worker to help her with this.

Further reading

Duncan, P (2010) *Values, Ethics and Health Care: Frameworks for Reasoning, Reflection and Debate.* London: SAGE.

This book is a useful reader for identifying the values and ethics which underpin healthcare and how these relate to learning.

Ellis, P, Engward, H and Howatson-Jones, L (2015) *Understanding Ethics for Nursing Students.* London: SAGE Publications.

This book sets out how ethics can be approached deductively and inductively and how students can use reflective techniques to enhance their ethical knowledge and understanding.

Hawley, G (2007) *Ethics in Clinical Practice: An Interprofessional Approach.* Harlow: Pearson Education.

This book is helpful for looking at shared ethical thinking and how this relates to practice.

Seedhouse, D (2009) *Ethics: The Heart of Healthcare,* 3rd edn. Chichester: John Wiley.

This book sets out ethical theory in an understandable manner.

Useful websites

www.nmc-uk.org

The website of the Nursing and Midwifery Council – where you can find a great deal of professional information including the latest guidance on the code of conduct for nurses and midwives.

www.gov.uk/government/policies/making-mental-health-services-more-effective-and-accessible-2
This website provides guidance to health and social care professionals on mental capacity issues and mental health services.

www.scie.org.uk/topic/careneeds/mentalhealth
The website for the Social Care Institute for Excellence has a page dedicated to mental health with information about government policies and best practice.

Chapter 9
Community health needs assessment

Susan Roberts

> 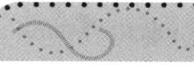 **NMC Standards for Pre-registration Nursing Education**
>
> This chapter will address the following competencies:
>
> **Domain 1: Professional values**
> 5. All nurses must fully understand the nurse's various roles, responsibilities and functions, and adapt their practice to meet the changing needs of people, groups, communities and populations.
>
> **Domain 2: Communication and interpersonal skills**
> 3. Nurses must promote the concept, knowledge and practice of self-care with people with acute and long-term conditions, using a range of communication skills and strategies.
>
> **Domain 3: Nursing practice and decision-making**
> 5. All nurses must understand public health principles, priorities and practice in order to recognise and respond to the major causes and social determinants of health, illness and health inequalities. They must use a range of information and data to assess the needs of people, groups, communities and populations, and work to improve health, well-being and experiences of healthcare; secure equal access to health screening, health promotion and healthcare; and promote social inclusion.
>
> **Domain 4: Leadership, management and team working**
> 1. All nurses must act as change agents and provide leadership through quality improvement and service development to enhance people's wellbeing and experiences of healthcare.

NMC Essential Skills Clusters (ESCs)

This chapter will address the following ESCs:

Cluster: Care, compassion and communication
1. As partners in the care process, people can trust a newly registered graduate nurse to provide collaborative care based on the highest standards, knowledge and competence.
2. People can trust the newly registered graduate nurse to engage in person-centred care empowering people to make choices about how their needs are met when they are unable to meet them for themselves.
4. People can trust a newly qualified graduate nurse to engage with them and their family or carers within their cultural environments in an acceptant and antidiscriminatory manner free from harassment and exploitation.

Cluster: Organisational aspects of care
10. People can trust the newly registered graduate nurse to deliver nursing interventions and evaluate their effectiveness against the agreed assessment and care plan.
18. People can trust a newly registered graduate nurse to enhance the safety of service users and identify and actively manage risk and uncertainty in relation to people, the environment, self and others.

Chapter aims

After reading this chapter you will be able to:

- explain what a community health needs assessment (CHNA) is and how it is developed;
- understand the policy context of CHNA;
- describe the differences between a CHNA and a health needs assessment (HNA) for a patient on an acute hospital ward;
- understand who is responsible for undertaking CHNAs and explain how to prepare and carry one out;
- explain the main benefits stemming from a CHNA to patients and practice.

Introduction

If you are to have an understanding of the wider picture of the assessment of health needs – and the subsequent planning and delivery of care to patients – it is important for you to explore CHNA. CHNA fits into the public health remit of community nurses and understanding it is an essential part of current nursing. The primary care (community) agenda and public health have been at the forefront of nursing practice for several years now. Public health is concerned with health issues affecting populations as well as individuals. It is also linked to health issues which may need to be addressed by bodies such as local health organisations, local authorities and, on the very broad scale, government departments. Community nurses have a very strong public health role (the history of which will be explored later in this chapter).

This chapter includes case studies from practice, each of which gives an example of innovations carried out as a direct result of what has been learned through a CHNA. In each case, the information from the CHNA led (through a decision-making process) to the planning and implementation of interventions which can be shown to have positive effects on achieving a higher level of wellness.

> **Case study: Practice example showing CHNA in action**
>
> *An example of how priorities are agreed and resources allocated can be seen in a project called Acorns, developed in Thurrock, Essex. This is a nurse-led project which provides wide-ranging services for refugees, asylum seekers, travelling families and homeless people – all groups that may not be registered with a GP. This project was developed by a health visitor (working with a public health focus), who became aware through her work that these groups of local people were experiencing difficulties accessing primary healthcare services such as GP services or baby clinics. As well as providing 'traditional' health services, the project provides other support such as filling in forms, and helps with language issues through the provision of interpreters in a variety of languages.*

Context and background: the beginnings of community nursing

Community nurses have a long history in caring for people in their own homes. They have always had a health promotion/education and public health function.

District nurses, health visitors and school nurses all have their roots in the Victorian public health movement. In 1859, district nursing services were set up in Liverpool to provide care for sick, poor people in their homes. Part of this care was offering nutritional and hygiene advice.

> **Activity 9.1** *Critical thinking*
>
> Florence Nightingale (1860) said *besides nursing the patient ... [this] shows them how they can call in sanitary help to make their one poor room more healthy.*
>
> The language used in this statement may sound strange, and even patronising, to modern ears. But consider carefully whether there are any similarities in the role of today's district nurses. Think particularly about health promotion and collaborative working.
>
> In 1862, the Manchester and Salford Ladies Sanitary Association employed women referred to as 'health visitors' to visit families in their own homes and offer advice on hygiene, sanitary and moral issues. Again, the terminology (for example, the word 'moral') may sound alien to us today, but can you see the beginnings of the modern-day health visitor?
>
> *An outline answer is given at the end of the chapter.*

Today, community nurses using CHNA continue and develop this Victorian tradition in adapting health services to meet the needs of people living in local communities. They address continuing social, demographic, environmental, political and economic change.

What is CHNA?

CHNA is an information-gathering exercise leading to an understanding of patterns of epidemiology (the study of patterns of disease) and demography (the study of populations). Factors such as age, gender, mortality rates (what people die from) and morbidity rates (what diseases people have) would be used. It also enables the identification of the major risk factors and causes of ill health, and enables the identification of the actions needed to address these (WHO, 2001). Information gained can be used to guide the delivery of appropriate and effective services to a community (Hogston and Marjoram, 2011). This is important because resources in the National Health Service are limited and effective planning is required in order to allocate them to the greatest effect. CHNA is a potentially powerful tool in enabling this process.

> ### Case study: Community initiative in Scotland
>
> *The following is an example of the health of the local community being improved as a direct result of carrying out a CHNA.*
>
> *Community nurses working in an area of Scotland carried out a CHNA by collecting information from the local community. The nurses gathered feedback and comments from a variety of sources:*
>
> - *individual patients they had been caring for;*
> - *questionnaires given out in the local community – in places such as mother and toddler groups, local pubs, youth clubs and to groups such as support networks for older people and the Women's Institute;*
> - *questionnaires displayed at local GP surgeries.*
>
> *The information gained in this way enabled the nurses to identify the priorities and concerns of the local population.*
>
> *From this information they identified groups of people living in a deprived inner-city estate who were interested in improving their health through healthier eating.*
>
> *These nurses helped to facilitate a gardening project (on disused land, and with the support of the local council) for participants to grow their own food. The produce was used by those actively involved and also sold to other local residents at affordable prices to encourage healthy eating in the community whilst also covering the costs of production. The community healthcare nurses facilitated the setting-up of this project using cross-department working and advocacy skills. Once the project was running successfully, the community nurses withdrew so that the residents could continue it themselves.*

> **Concept summary**
>
> CHNA is a broad multifaceted process which has many functions.
>
> - CHNA examines the state of the health of the local population.
> - CHNA explores the factors affecting the health of the local population.
> - CHNA identifies potential risk factors affecting the health of the population.
> - CHNA plans strategies to address these risk factors.

Looking at current nursing practice, the Royal College of Nursing (2012) highlights the aims of nursing services delivering public health as being to:

- increase life expectancy by influencing healthy behaviours;
- reduce health inequalities, for example, targeting vulnerable populations to improve health outcomes and access services;
- improve population health, for example, reducing obesity and alcohol abuse, improving sexual health behaviour;
- increase the awareness of positive healthy behaviours in communities;
- promote and develop social capital;
- engage with individuals, families and communities to influence the design and development of services.

CHNA	HNA in a hospital setting
Not specifically disease-focused	Relates to the presenting medical problem
Proactive (seeking out health needs)	Predominantly reactive (while looking at actual and potential problems)
Utilises a public health model	Utilises a variety of nursing models
Has a clear focus on health and aims to enable a higher level of wellness	Focuses on both health and illness and aims to enable a higher level of wellness
Deals with known and unknown need	Largely deals with what is known need and potentially may not have an awareness of what is unknown need

Table 9.1: A comparison between community health needs assessment (CHNA) and health needs assessment (HNA)

Source: adapted from Gillam et al., 2007.

The Department of Health (2010) defines CHNA *as a systematic method for reviewing the health issues facing a population, leading to agreed priorities and resource allocation that will improve health and reduce inequalities.* It differs from HNA in a hospital setting in several important ways, as shown in Table 9.1.

Why you need to know about CHNA

You will need to understand what a CHNA is and how it works because, as a nurse working in any setting (community/hospital/nursing home/clinic), your patients have lives, families, homes, 'worlds' which have a direct impact on their health. Your patients' community background has a profound influence on their health. For instance, if a person lives in a very damp, cold house, this could contribute directly to a severe chest infection from pneumonia, resulting in admission to hospital.

The patient's community/home background certainly has a profound impact in relation to discharge planning. A CHNA would enable the nurses in the patient's community to have a clear picture of the health needs of that community/population and to focus planned activities and resources to address these. For instance, in the case of the patient admitted to hospital with pneumonia, a CHNA would enable the community nurses to access local community projects/ initiatives which can help him to find funding for insulating his house. These initiatives/projects may be carried out by local charities or voluntary groups. The wide and in-depth local community knowledge gained from the CHNA can give the community nurses detailed knowledge of any suitable projects as well as providing them with links to a broad network of useful colleagues across a very wide range of sectors (the voluntary sector, charities, local housing departments) as well as social services.

With good team work between the hospital nurses and the community nurses, it may be possible for some of this work to be planned or started before the patient is discharged.

Activity 9.2 — Critical thinking

Think about a patient you have cared for in hospital whose health had almost certainly been affected by the circumstances in which he or she lived in the community.

If you were planning this patient's discharge from hospital, what factors would you need to take into consideration? What information would you hope might be available to you from a CHNA in order to ensure that discharge planning for this patient was aimed at ensuring the patient would be able to remain in good health once back in the community?

An outline answer is given at the end of the chapter.

We will explore more practice examples of how CHNA can work throughout this chapter.

CHNA as an assessment process

When carrying out an assessment on an individual, you might use a model such as Roper, Logan and Tierney's activities of daily living (ADL; see Chapter 7: Roper et al., 2000) and look at aspects such as mobility and breathing. When carrying out a CHNA you would be carrying out a similarly holistic assessment on a community, using a framework/model (such as the five-step approach described later in this chapter), and assessing aspects affecting health, such as public transport services and mobility. Not all of the ADLs have such a clear link with aspects of a CHNA, but there are obvious corollaries between some, such as breathing and pollution levels.

The process of CHNA is structured along similar lines to an individual assessment, looking at the community rather as if it were a whole person.

> **Activity 9.3** *Critical thinking*
>
> Look at an example of assessment documentation based on Roper, Logan and Tierney's ADL model. Can you make any other connections (such as the example of breathing and pollution levels) between the individual assessment of the ADLs and possible areas you might assess in the community as part of a CHNA?
>
> *An outline answer is given at the end of the chapter.*

Why is CHNA useful?

CHNA is used to plan and deliver the most effective care to those in greatest need. It enables the nurse to work in collaboration with the population and other professionals and organisations to bring about maximum health benefits effectively.

> **Activity 9.4** *Reflection*
>
> In some areas of healthcare, services can be seen to be driven by the priorities of the professionals or the service, as opposed to being needs-led.
>
> As healthcare professionals, do you think we always have the same views as our patients and the general public as to what is a priority? Reflect on an instance in your own practice where this has perhaps not been the case.
>
> *An outline answer is given at the end of the chapter.*

The NHS Plan (Department of Health, 2000) laid out a firm intention that the views of the public ought to be at the heart of healthcare planning. It aimed to create a service that was geared around the views and priorities of the patients, service users and public. Patients and members of the public were invited to take part in local forums where local health issues were discussed. Patients' views were to be taken into account on decisions such as how money would be spent by local health services.

Following on from that, in 2006 the Department of Health carried out an extensive consultation exercise, involving 42,861 people in total, seeking out their views on what they considered to be priorities in health and how to improve health services provided in the community. This consultation process resulted in the document *Your Health, Your Care, Your Say* (Department of Health, 2006). One of the recommendations that came out of this listening exercise was to extend GP opening hours.

CHNA is embedded in government policy as part of its aim to reduce health inequalities (NICE, 2005). Reducing inequalities in healthcare could be seen as aiming towards a fair system of healthcare provision as well as producing more positive outcomes and being more responsive to change (Sines et al., 2009).

In recent health and social care policy, the importance of accurately targeting services (and resources) in a bespoke manner has been further highlighted (NHS England, 2014). There is a need to tailor make services appropriate to the specific needs of a community, as opposed to a 'one size fits all' approach. Examples of this strategy in action could be an option where community nurses work with other community specialists, social care professionals, mental health nurses, GPs and hospital specialists to create integrated out-of-hospital care (the Multispeciality Provider) (NHS England, 2014). Examples of this could include multi professional/multi agency (including the voluntary sector) on projects such as food banks. Such an innovative way of working would clearly rely on accurate local data – provided by a CHNA.

In healthcare terms equity refers to the idea of fairness, where we are attempting to get rid of unfair differences in provision of services across differing socioeconomic or geographical groups. This issue has been an important aspect of primary care since the Alma Ata declaration of 1978 (World Health Organization, United Nations' Children's Fund, 1978). Social justice again incorporates the idea of fairness; for instance, aiming for services for teenagers or the elderly to be of similar standards regardless of geographical location or income.

CHNA can be used as part of a planning cycle, informing local plans to meet local needs. It is an important first step in planning health strategies for a community, meeting health needs and planning health promotion activities. This process can enable nurses to make these activities relevant and effective, leading to positive outcomes and health benefits for patients.

Case study: Carers in the community

Using the information gathered for the local profile, one group of community nurses identified (from local GP practice data) a significantly high percentage of older people with dementia living in the area – an isolated country setting. As a result, the community psychiatric nurse team working with older people in the locality liaised with the practice nurses across the identified GP practices with a view to improving the provision of support for the carers involved. This involved linking in with voluntary groups to provide transport to pick up carers and take them to support group meetings, and also with agencies to provide respite care.

Who carries out a CHNA?

Activity 9.5 — Reflection

If you have already had a community placement, think back to the range of professionals you came across.

Reflect back on your own experiences.

- Did you understand their roles?
- Did you see CHNA being carried out or discussed?
- Who was involved in this information-gathering exercise?
- Who do you think should have been involved?
- Do you think professionals should work together in this exercise?

If you are about to have a community placement, think about these issues when you go out.

This is your own reflection, therefore no outline answer is provided.

Exactly who is involved in carrying out this process may vary considerably in different locations. Ideally, CHNA should be carried out as a collaborative team effort in order to avoid duplication of information and to benefit from a range of relevant and appropriate expertise and stances.

Traditionally CHNA was seen as the health visitor's responsibility. However it is now firmly in government policy as part of the role of all community nurses. This reflects the evolution of community nurses.

Case study: Collaboration across communities

One project developed from a group of district nurses carrying out a CHNA. From profiling the area covered by a local GP practice, community nurses identified a high incidence of falls in older people in the catchment area. This information inspired them to set up a programme of regular falls prevention sessions in the local community hall, linking in with national policies on falls prevention.

Working in a collaborative manner to carry out a CHNA requires nurses to have excellent communication skills. It demands vigilant attention to issues such as data protection and storage of information. It can also be a fertile and productive way of trying out innovative ways of working – for instance, community nurses from different specialties working together in a more integrated way, challenging traditional, restrictive boundaries.

> **Case study: An inspirational example of innovative and collaborative working from a student nurse**
>
> *An example of collaborative working and innovative ways of working can be seen in a project set up by a student nurse in Chester. Louise Williamson had some experiences of volunteering with various community groups. She then initiated the setting up of 'Treehouse', a food kitchen aimed at people who were homeless and/or those with social and economic problems. Louise worked in partnership with local organisations such as local church groups and The Samaritans. The project not only provides meals and hot drinks, but also provides a safe warm environment and the opportunity for social interaction with others. It also provides links and advice on other services including housing and employment (www.chester.ac.uk/node/27691).*

How to go about preparing for a CHNA

In order to gain a clear and full picture of all the various factors in the area which may have an impact on the health of the community, the community nursing team needs a wide range of information. However, exactly what information might be most relevant will vary from one area to another, as will the way it is collected. Activity 9.6 is designed to get you thinking about where to start. You might find it particularly helpful if you work alongside one or more colleagues and spend some time discussing your findings and thinking about how and why they may be different.

> **Activity 9.6** *Decision-making*
>
> If you were a community nurse, what information do you think you would need in order to carry out a CHNA? What would you measure? Think broadly of all the factors in a community that would give you valuable information relevant to the health needs of the people living in that area. Make a list and discuss with a colleague.
>
> Now think about the area you live in. How would you find out the information you have identified in Activity 9.6? What would be your sources of information? Who might you need to contact to find out some of the information?
>
> Once again, you will get more out of this activity if you write down your findings and discuss with one or more colleagues.
>
> *An outline answer is given at the end of the chapter.*

The vital role of the community nurse in assessing the health needs of a community is highlighted by the RCN, which identifies the need for nurses to be 'actively engaged and looking for those at risk of major preventable health issues' (RCN, 2012, p13). They add that community nurses need to 'identify high incidence of hospital readmissions, seek out the cause and target vulnerable populations' (RCN, 2012, p13). The RCN describes this concept as 'upstreaming' – a very accessible term to visualise these community nursing activities – which involves pre-empting problems (seeking out the causes of problems and attempting to prevent them) and stopping them from progressing further 'downstream'.

A five-step structured approach to CHNA

Once you have explored some of the background issues through Activity 9.6, you can start to think about structuring your approach to CHNA. There are many different practical frameworks for undertaking this exercise. A five-step process, such as that advocated by NICE (2005), is a useful place to start, and Figure 9.1 shows how that might work in practice.

Step 1 starts with identifying the population – for example, is it the nurse's caseload, or a geographical area, or are you looking at the population defined by the caseload of a GP/group of GPs with whom the community nurses work? Step 1 also defines your aims. Are you aiming to try and address areas of great health need in your area (e.g. falls in the elderly)? What could be the risks if you are not successful, having raised expectations you were unable to meet, for example?

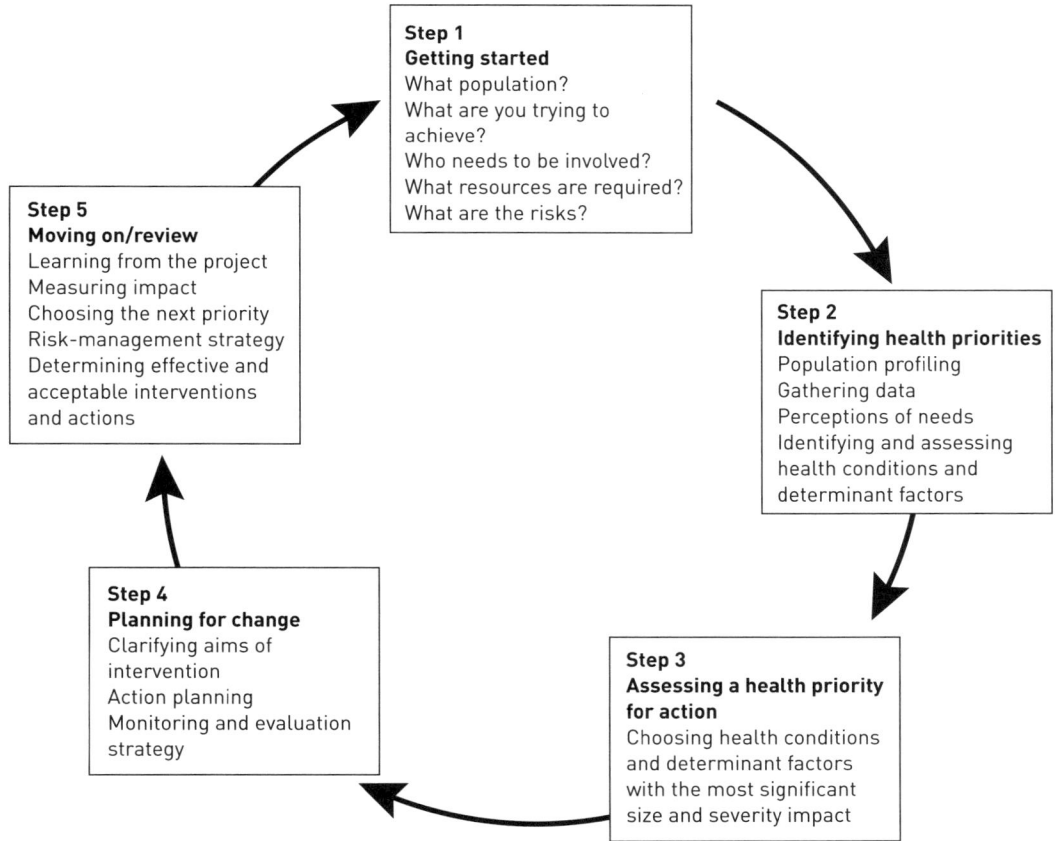

Figure 9.1: Community health needs assessment as a cyclical, dynamic process

Step 2 involves searching out information from a range of sources, such as the census, Director of Public Health reports, GP practice database, local government information (for instance, on housing and pollution). It also requires an understanding of the concept of need: whose perspective or view of priorities are you using?

Step 3 involves analysing the data and identifying priorities. What are the major health needs in the area? Is there a high rate of unplanned teenage pregnancies, for example, or a high number of toddlers having accidents? Is there poverty resulting in referrals from care professionals to food banks? (You might like to look at the statistics of the Trussell Trust which show a tripling of food bank use year on year since 2012: available from: **www.trusselltrust.org/stats**).

When you reach step 4, you will be putting the plans into action. What are you going to do about the needs you have identified? Who will be involved in any projects? What resources will you need? How will you evaluate the project and measure whether you have been successful?

In step 5 you are evaluating, reflecting back on the experience and then planning to go through the cycle again, taking account of any new information. You may discover that, for example, your new system of teenage health drop-in clinics at a local gym has been evaluated by the participants as being very positive. You might therefore want to continue with this or even expand it. This may involve seeking out further sources of funding.

As Figure 9.1 demonstrates, the process of carrying out a CHNA should be a cyclical, dynamic one, not a one-off series of actions. This has implications for the use of community nurses' time, and is another argument for carrying out the process as a collaborative exercise. Various different combinations of community nurses sometimes work together to produce a CHNA, e.g. there may be a health visitor, district nurse, practice nurse and community psychiatric nurse, all of whom work with a similar population and geographical area who would collaborate to produce the CHNA, rather than each of them working separately, therefore avoiding potentially duplicating work.

Before you start the next activity it would be useful to look at the terms 'prevalence' and 'incidence'. You may have come across these terms before: they are defined in the box below.

> **Concept summary: Prevalence and incidence**
>
> - Prevalence is 'the number of existing cases in a defined population at a defined point in time, divided by the total number of people in that population at the same point in time' (Carnerio and Howard, 2011, p18). For instance, 'The prevalence of breast cancer in a small rural village in Wales in June 2011 was 0.01'. This number can never be more than one.
> - Incidence is 'the frequency of new (incident) cases in a defined population during a specified time period' (Carnerio and Howard, 2011, p18). For example, 'There were two new cases of breast cancer in a small rural village in Wales between June and August 2011'.
>
> Prevalence, then, is looking at the full picture of the total number of cases at any one time, where incidence is looking at the number of new cases.

> The concepts of prevalence and incidence could be described as 'Disease distribution' (Aschengrau and Seage, 2013). Disease distribution involves the analysis of a variety of characteristics of the disease, that is to say the Who? Where? and When? Examining these characteristics can help us to understand the health status of a population and then plan and implement appropriate strategies (Aschengrau and Seage, 2013).

Activity 9.7 — Research and evidence-based practice

Find a copy of the Director of Public Health report from one of the following:

www.apho.org.uk
www.dh.gov.uk (this website will be useful in other contexts too)
www.kmpho.nhs.uk
www.newcastle.gov.uk/health-and-social-care/health-services/public-health-annual-report

OR

Look at the report in your own local area, or the website of the trust where you are on placement.

Choose one of the following categories:

- older people living at home with chronic diseases;
- teenage pregnancies;
- reducing the levels of substance and alcohol misuse;
- deaths from heart disease.

Look at the assessment that was carried out, and focus particularly on the part that relates to your chosen category.

Now try to answer the following questions:

- What is the incidence within one community?
- What is the prevalence within this community?

Looking at the decision-making:

Is there evidence of strategies addressing the issues?
What are examples of current service provision to address the needs?
What decisions would you have made (based on the assessments) to address the needs?

This activity does not have an outline answer as it is based on your own research.

The real-life examples we have looked at in this chapter should give you an idea of the range of ways in which information gained from a CHNA can be used, and inspire you to look at some of the many and varied community health innovations and initiatives that may be carried out in practice in your area.

> **Activity 9.8** *Communication*
>
> Try to find some examples of community health innovations in the area where you live. You may see articles in your local press, or advertised in your GP practice. When you go out on a community placement, talk to your mentor about CHNA in his or her practice and any activities your mentor is involved with as a result.
>
> *This activity does not have an outline answer as it is based on your own experience.*

Conclusion

All nurses have a responsibility for improving the health of the public. It is important to be aware that, in order to achieve this, a multidisciplinary approach is vital. The factors that potentially have an impact on the health of the public are not exclusively within the realm and remit of health professionals. The wide spectrum of factors impacting on health need to be incorporated into any strategies to improve health – we need to keep in mind the 'bigger picture'. In order to be able to incorporate these factors into planning care for our patients and the public, we need firstly to identify what the factors are: what is the 'bigger picture'? CHNA is an effective method of assessing this.

> **Chapter summary**
>
> We have explored how CHNA plays a central role in community nursing practice. It is a vital aspect of the assessment and decision-making required by community nurses, and is an ongoing, logical and cyclical process. The assessment carried out in this manner leads naturally on to decision-making processes, which then lead to action in response.
>
> We looked at how CHNA is a fundamentally important area of community nursing, emanating as it does from the public health roots of the profession. It is also an important area for all nurses to be aware of as part of the 'bigger picture' affecting all patients.
>
> We have identified that the ethos of CHNA is in line with both patient-centredness and the principles of primary care. It incorporates concepts of patient empowerment and collaboration, respecting autonomy. The process aims to address issues of inequalities and exclusion.

Activities: brief outline answers

Activity 9.1 Critical thinking [page 123]

Modern district nurses still visit patients in their own homes, providing both holistic care and health promotion advice. In order to fulfil this role they work in collaboration with a wide range of other professionals and groups across not just the health and social care spectrum. For instance, district nurses may sometimes need to contact the local housing department, acting as the patient's advocate, regarding improvements to the patient's housing situation (such as a damp flat or windows in need of repair).

Health visitors also still make home visits to children and families (as well as clinic work) and provide a range of supportive and health-monitoring services. They provide health promotion advice and offer support to families about child welfare and care.

Activity 9.2 Critical thinking [page 126]

While the patient is on your ward, a discharge-planning process would be carried out. This process should ideally begin when the patient is admitted, or even earlier in the case of planned admissions (DH, 2010). As part of this process, the ward multidisciplinary team would be carrying out assessments looking at all aspects that may affect the patient's safe discharge. This would include their home living conditions. These assessments may reveal that there are aspects of these home conditions that may have a detrimental effect on the patient's health – for instance, that the patient's house is damp. Good communication between the hospital and community staff may enable improvements or adjustments to be made to the patient's house before the patient is discharged.

Activity 9.3 Critical thinking [page 127]

Some other examples of where the ADLs in a hospital assessment of an individual patient may have clear links to aspects community nurses may have identified from the CHNA might be:

- controlling temperature – What is the general condition of housing in the community? Are there a lot of old neglected rental properties without central heating or insulation?
- maintaining a safe environment – Are there busy roads in the community? Are there enough safe places to cross roads? Are there adequate safe footpaths and street lighting?
- working and playing – What is the general level of employment/unemployment in the community? What are the local leisure facilities like? Are there public parks, cycle paths, public swimming baths and libraries?
- sleeping – What are the levels of noise like at night? For example, is there excessive traffic noise, or noise from industrial activities?

Activity 9.4 Reflection [page 127]

An example of this potential difference in priorities may be illustrated by the following anecdote. A practice nurse is carrying out blood pressure checks in a local supermarket. She discovers that Mr X has blood pressure of 200/120mmHg. She then tries to interest Mr X in an action plan to address this. The practice nurse's priority is for Mr X to reduce his blood pressure to within acceptable limits. Mr X had actually walked into the supermarket to do his shopping after work feeling perfectly well and with no idea at all that there was anything wrong with his blood pressure. He is, however, extremely worried about the fact that he and his wife desperately want to have a baby and are having trouble conceiving. This is his priority.

Activity 9.6 Decision making [page 130]

What information do you need? What would you measure?

Remember you would be trying to create a full, holistic assessment of the community, so you would be assessing a wide range of factors. The table below may be helpful as a reminder.

Factor for assessment	Aspects to be taken into account
Housing	How much is rented?
Public or private landlord?	What is the general condition of housing like?
Public transport	Do the local transport facilities serve the needs of the population?
	Are they suitable for mothers and babies/elderly or disabled people?

professionals and groups across not just the health and social care spectrum. For instance, district nurses may sometimes need to contact the local housing department, acting as the patient's advocate, regarding improvements to the patient's housing situation (such as a damp flat or windows in need of repair).

Health visitors also still make home visits to children and families (as well as clinic work) and provide a range of supportive and health-monitoring services. They provide health promotion advice and offer support to families about child welfare and care.

Activity 9.2 Critical thinking [page 126]

While the patient is on your ward, a discharge-planning process would be carried out. This process should ideally begin when the patient is admitted, or even earlier in the case of planned admissions (DH, 2010). As part of this process, the ward multidisciplinary team would be carrying out assessments looking at all aspects that may affect the patient's safe discharge. This would include their home living conditions. These assessments may reveal that there are aspects of these home conditions that may have a detrimental effect on the patient's health – for instance, that the patient's house is damp. Good communication between the hospital and community staff may enable improvements or adjustments to be made to the patient's house before the patient is discharged.

Activity 9.3 Critical thinking [page 127]

Some other examples of where the ADLs in a hospital assessment of an individual patient may have clear links to aspects community nurses may have identified from the CHNA might be:

- controlling temperature – What is the general condition of housing in the community? Are there a lot of old neglected rental properties without central heating or insulation?
- maintaining a safe environment – Are there busy roads in the community? Are there enough safe places to cross roads? Are there adequate safe footpaths and street lighting?
- working and playing – What is the general level of employment/unemployment in the community? What are the local leisure facilities like? Are there public parks, cycle paths, public swimming baths and libraries?
- sleeping – What are the levels of noise like at night? For example, is there excessive traffic noise, or noise from industrial activities?

Activity 9.4 Reflection [page 127]

An example of this potential difference in priorities may be illustrated by the following anecdote. A practice nurse is carrying out blood pressure checks in a local supermarket. She discovers that Mr X has blood pressure of 200/120mmHg. She then tries to interest Mr X in an action plan to address this. The practice nurse's priority is for Mr X to reduce his blood pressure to within acceptable limits. Mr X had actually walked into the supermarket to do his shopping after work feeling perfectly well and with no idea at all that there was anything wrong with his blood pressure. He is, however, extremely worried about the fact that he and his wife desperately want to have a baby and are having trouble conceiving. This is his priority.

Activity 9.6 Decision making [page 130]

What information do you need? What would you measure?

Remember you would be trying to create a full, holistic assessment of the community, so you would be assessing a wide range of factors. The table below may be helpful as a reminder.

Factor for assessment	Aspects to be taken into account
Housing	How much is rented?
Public or private landlord?	What is the general condition of housing like?
Public transport	Do the local transport facilities serve the needs of the population?
	Are they suitable for mothers and babies/elderly or disabled people?

(Continued)

Factor for assessment	Aspects to be taken into account
Employment/unemployment	Are there unemployment levels that may be causing socioeconomic deprivation?
Air pollution levels	Are these acceptable? Are they a potential health hazard?
Crime rates	Are these a cause of anxiety for housebound people, for example?
Education	Educational achievement levels: Do local schools/colleges have good results on the league tables? Does this have potential implications for employment opportunities?
Epidemiology and patterns of disease	Morbidity – what diseases are people in the local area being affected by? Mortality – what are people dying from and when?
Demography	What are the numbers in different age ranges and gender patterns within the local population?

How would you find this information? What sources would you use? Who might you need to contact?

There is a wide variety of sources to provide you with all this information, such as the census results; Director of Public Health reports; Environmental Health Office; reports from the Department of Education; and GP practice data.

Further reading

Chilton, S, Bain, H, Clarridge, A and Melling, K (2012) *Textbook of Community Nursing.* London: Hodder Arnold.

This has some useful case studies.

Hubley, J and Copeman, J (2008) *Practical Health Promotion.* Cambridge: Polity.

This has a good section on assessing health in the community.

Useful websites

www.nhs.uk/ServiceDirectories/Pages/GP.aspx?pid=0846D25C-8F05-408A-8CD6-A9E809069C49

This website will give you a rich variety of examples of CHNA being used to improve health in the community, in the Acorns project.

www.gov.uk/government/organisations/public-health-england

This website is a good way to keep up to date with new public health developments, including issues related to nursing roles and innovations.

Chapter 10
Patient assessment and decision-making

Mooi Standing

NMC Standards for Pre-registration Nursing Education

This chapter will address the following competencies:

Domain 1: Professional values
9. All nurses must appreciate the value of evidence in practice, be able to understand and appraise research, apply relevant theory and research findings to their work, and identify areas for further investigation.

Domain 2: Communication and interpersonal skills
5. All nurses must recognise and respond effectively, using therapeutic principles, to people who are anxious or in distress in order to promote wellbeing and manage personal safety. They must know when other specialist interventions may be needed, including independent advocacy services, and make the referral.

Domain 3: Nursing practice and decision-making
1. All nurses must work closely with individuals, groups and carers, using a range of skills to carry out comprehensive, systematic and holistic assessments. These must take into account current and previous physical, social, cultural, psychological, spiritual, genetic and environmental factors that may be relevant to the individual and their families.
2. All nurses must listen, recognise and respond to an individual's physical, social and psychological needs. They must plan, deliver and evaluate technically safe, competent, person-centred care that addresses all their daily activities, in partnership with people and their carers, families and other professionals.
7. All nurses must know when a person of any age is at risk and in a vulnerable situation in any environment and in need of extra support and protection. They must also act to safeguard them against abuse of any kind.

Domain 4: Leadership, management and team working
9. All nurses must work within local policy to assess and manage risk effectively, reporting risk and raising concerns while maintaining the rights, wellbeing, security and safety of everyone involved in the care process.

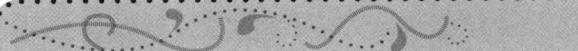

NMC Essential Skills Clusters

This chapter will address the following ESCs:

Cluster: Care, compassion and communication

4. People can trust a newly qualified graduate nurse to engage with them and their family or carers within their cultural environments in an acceptant and antidiscriminatory manner free from harassment and exploitation.

By the first progression point:

5. Evaluates ways in which own interactions affect relationships to ensure that they do not impact inappropriately on others.

By entry to the register:

7. Manages and defuses challenging situations effectively.

Cluster: Organisational aspects of care

11. People can trust the newly registered graduate nurse to safeguard children and adults from vulnerable situations and support and protect them from harm.

By the second progression point:

4. Document concerns and information about people who are in vulnerable situations.

By entry to register:

5. Recognises and responds when people are in vulnerable situations and at risk, or in need of support and protection.

Chapter aims

After reading this chapter you will be able to:

- describe how patient assessment influences clinical decisions and interventions;
- appreciate the uncertainties, challenges and changing nature of health problems;
- identify strengths and weaknesses of intuitive versus analytical clinical judgement;
- apply cognitive continuum theory – nine modes of practice – to assessment and care;
- apply a matrix model – ten perceptions of decision-making – to assessment and care;
- apply a 'PERSON' evaluation tool to assessment and decision-making in nursing care.

Introduction

Without accurate assessment of health problems, any decisions made about a person's care are likely to be unsafe and ineffective. Assessment, clinical judgement and decision-making are therefore closely linked because accurate identification of health problems needs to go hand in hand with delivering safe and effective nursing interventions. Chapters 1–9 showed how assessment involves gathering relevant information from various sources (e.g. what patients tell you, research evidence) in order to diagnose health problems, and then plan ethical, holistic nursing care (for individuals and communities) to address the problems. Using case studies, this chapter relates assessment of health problems to the clinical judgement, decision-making and interventions used to tackle them. Relevant theory and research including cognitive continuum theory – nine modes of practice – and a matrix model – ten perceptions of clinical decision-making (Standing, 2010, 2014) – are applied to patient assessment. Finally, a 'PERSON' evaluation tool (Standing, 2014), developed in response to criticisms of nursing practice in the Francis Report (2013), is applied to review and enhance patient assessment and decision-making in nursing.

Assessment, clinical judgement, decision-making and healthcare interventions

The following case study highlights the interrelationship between assessment, clinical judgement, decision-making and nursing/interprofessional healthcare interventions.

Case study: Assessing Angela's ear complaint and deciding what to do about it

Angela, age 48, is a police chief inspector. Part of her personal hygiene regime involves cleaning the inside of her ears with cotton buds. There are signs on the packaging warning against inserting them in ears but Angela feels uncomfortable when she senses her ears need cleaning and this is the best method she has found to do so. One day a cotton bud detaches itself and gets stuck inside her left ear. In trying to get it out Angela pushes it further inside, increasing her discomfort. She takes paracetamol tablets every four hours to help control the pain.

Two days later Angela cannot bear the constant irritation and pain any more so goes to see her GP. He uses an auroscope to examine her ear and sees the bud but is unable to remove it. He refers Angela to the practice nurse (trained in electrical ear irrigation) for the removal of a 'foreign body' in her left ear. However, the device is in need of repair and so the nurse advises Angela to go to the local minor injury unit (MIU).

Kim is a first-year nursing student observing Nigel, a nurse practitioner at the MIU, who sits behind a desk in the consulting room while Angela explains what the problem is. Nigel gets up, examines her ear with an auroscope, but cannot see anything that should not be there. Kim notices that Angela is getting irritated when she says, 'It has been there for the last two days. It is hurting my ear. It's making me feel dizzy and I cannot concentrate on my work. My GP saw it this morning and said it could be removed, so if you are unable to see it, surely you can still irrigate the ear and then it might come out?'

Kim senses that Nigel might feel that his competence is being challenged. He asks Angela whether the GP used an auroscope like he did to examine her. An argument ensues as Angela champions the GP's expertise, Nigel claims that he is also a qualified medical practitioner, and Angela retorts that he is a nurse, not a doctor. Kim feels torn between respecting her senior colleague and sensing that Angela is not well.

continued ...

> *Nigel asks Helen, a nurse practitioner colleague, to examine Angela's ear (using an auroscope) and she states that she can see no foreign object. Nigel tells Angela they can find nothing wrong so they will not be irrigating her ear. Angela leaves the MIU (after filling in an evaluation form where she is very critical of the care received) feeling very frustrated because she does not feel any better but has been told there is nothing wrong. She contacts the surgery and is offered an urgent appointment with a different GP. He cannot see any foreign body, but he notices that the ear is very inflamed, prescribes antibiotics (by mouth) and refers Angela to an ear, nose and throat (ENT) clinic. The ENT consultant confirms there is no foreign body in her left ear ('the cotton bud must have fallen out') but that her ear remains infected. He informs Angela that ear irrigation is not recommended for ear infections, and prescribes antibiotic ear drops. He advises Angela not to use cotton buds any more but to use wax-softening ear drops to clean her ears in future. One week later Angela feels much better.*

Angela's case study shows how a seemingly innocuous event like a cotton bud getting stuck in a person's ear can result in pain, discomfort, irritability and infection (which if not treated could cause more serious problems, e.g. deafness). The case study also conveys how many people can be involved in one person's care in a short space of time, and the variations in their assessment of the health problem and what they did about it. Activity 10.1 gives you a structure to guide your reflection about Angela's case study so that you can appreciate some of the challenges and uncertainties of patient assessment and related healthcare interventions.

Activity 10.1 — *Critical thinking*

The purpose of this activity is to get you involved in exploring some of the issues discussed, identifying different ways that Angela's problem was assessed and treated, and for you to become more aware of the interrelationships between assessment, clinical judgement and decision-making. Read the case study again and then complete the following table by summarising how each person diagnosed (defined) the problem and what action they decided to take to resolve the problem.

Angela's case study

Person doing assessment	Problems they identified	Their decision-making/action
Angela		
First GP		
Practice nurse		
Nigel (nurse practitioner)		
Helen (nurse practitioner)		
Kim (student nurse)		

Patient assessment and decision-making

Second GP		
ENT consultant		

An outline answer is given at the end of the chapter.

Activity 10.1 brings to light some challenges and uncertainties in trying to reach an accurate diagnosis of a health problem and deciding the best course of action to take. In Angela's case study, the varied assessments and related clinical decision-making fall into three main groups, as shown in Table 10.1.

	Assessment and diagnosis	Clinical decision-making and action
1	Cotton bud/foreign body in left ear causing pain and discomfort	Remove foreign body from left ear
2	No foreign body in left ear and no health problem evident	No treatment required
3	Inflammation and infection in left ear causing pain and discomfort	Prescribe antibiotics to kill the bacteria causing the infection and thereby relieve symptoms

Table 10.1: Assessments and resulting decision-making

Each person assessing Angela's health problem used information (e.g. from what Angela reported, general observations and examination of her left ear) to make a decision based on the evidence available to them. The fact that they reached different diagnoses enables us to reach the following conclusions.

- Assessment, clinical judgement and decision-making are not an exact science.
- Healthcare practitioners have different sets of skills and may view problems differently.
- The potential for them to make errors means that nurses and doctors need to assess risks carefully regarding their proposed interventions (e.g. Nigel missed signs of infection but he was right not to irrigate the ear when he saw no reason to because irrigation, although safer than ear syringing, can sometimes cause damage, especially if the ear is infected).
- Health problems are not static: they can clear up, stay the same, get worse or change (e.g. the cotton bud causing discomfort apparently fell out but Angela still had an ear infection).
- Due to their changeable nature, health problems need to be continuously reassessed so that clinical judgement, decision-making and related interventions can be adjusted if need be.

Chapter 10

A flow chart rounds off this section, summarising the interrelationships between assessment of problems, diagnosis, clinical judgement, decision-making and healthcare interventions (Figure 10.1). In Activity 10.2 you are asked to discuss and apply this flow chart to clinical practice.

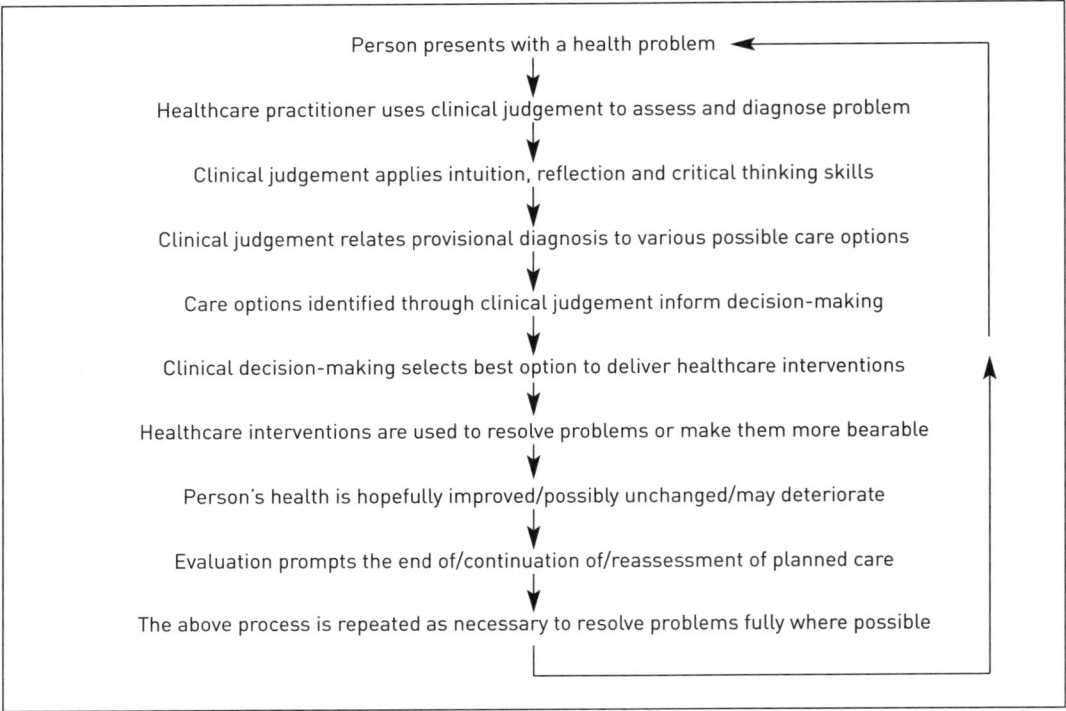

Figure 10.1: Assessment, clinical judgement, decision-making and healthcare interventions

Activity 10.2 — Reflection and teamwork

The aim of this activity is to reinforce your understanding of the interrelationships between assessment, diagnosis, clinical judgement, decision-making and healthcare interventions. It also encourages you to appreciate teamwork in assessment and clinical decision-making. Get together with some colleagues and work through the flow chart (Figure 10.1) thinking of examples from your combined experiences of practice placements. Remember how in Angela's case study, many different health professionals were involved, so try to incorporate the contributions of everyone concerned in the examples of patient assessment you and your colleagues identify. See if you can tease out different ways that they may have diagnosed a person's health problem and any differences in their clinical decision-making and interventions. Reflect on why this might have been so with reference to the various types of evidence on which they may have based their clinical judgement and decision-making. Review the effectiveness of interventions used in terms of patient outcomes, and how this influenced subsequent clinical decision-making. Finally, reflect on what you have learned from the activity and what aspects of the process described in the flow chart you feel you

> need to learn more about. See if you and your colleagues can help each other understand any issues a little better and/or agree plans to find out more.
>
> As this activity is for you and your colleagues to discuss and learn from, no outline answer is given.

Applying decision theory and research to patient assessment and healthcare

Standing (2010) applied cognitive continuum theory to nursing/healthcare using nine modes of practice (mentioned in Chapter 2), used now to review decisions in Angela's case study.

Nine modes	Examples of decision-making in Angela's case study of practice
Intuitive judgement	Angela felt it was OK to use cotton buds to clean her ear despite warnings against doing so; Kim sensed that Angela was not well when she became irritated
Reflective judgement	Kim reflected on feeling torn between respecting senior colleague Nigel and empathising with Angela
Patient and peer-aided judgement	Angela explained the problem to practitioners and described her symptoms (e.g. pain); they referred Angela to other practitioners (e.g. Nigel asked Helen to examine the ear)
System-aided judgement	Special equipment (auroscope) used to examine ears; systematic problem-solving approach adopted by all
Critical review of experiential and research evidence	Angela was critical of the care she received in the MIU; the second GP and ENT consultant recognised signs of infection and knew which antibiotics to prescribe as treatment
Action research and clinical audit	Angela completed an evaluation form in the MIU to give feedback on aspects of care that she felt were poor; faulty electrical ear irrigation device needs repair at surgery; ENT consultant advises Angela to stop putting cotton buds in her ears and to clean them with ear drops instead
Qualitative research	Angela's experience of care is a qualitative case study; Kim's reflections on what she has learned from her experiences could be written up and published one day
Survey research	Review of electrical ear irrigation indicates it is safer than ear syringing but it still carries risks (e.g. damaging the ear drum if pressure is excessive or causing infection)
Experimental research	The antibiotics prescribed are developed and tested through scientific research and clinical trials

Table 10.2: Nine modes of practice applied to Angela's case study

As you can see above, each of the nine modes of practice can be applied to review the decisions referred to in Angela's case study. This shows the wide range of knowledge and evidence that nurses and other practitioners draw upon in their clinical judgement and decision-making. Cognitive continuum theory of judgement and decision-making combines the two opposing extremes of *intuitive human judgement* which is informed by a person's own subjective experience versus *analytical decision-making* which is informed by objective, scientific research (Hammond, 1996). The nine modes of practice show how judgement and decision-making can contain varying amounts of intuition and analysis ranging from a 'gut feeling' about someone to giving medicine developed by scientific research and clinical trials.

Ideally, you don't have a favourite mode of practice that you stick to regardless of the circumstances. Intuition is invaluable when you have to make 'on the spot' decisions to react quickly when necessary but if you rely too much on intuition, you are likely to ignore important research evidence (e.g. Angela ignored the warning not to put a cotton bud in her ear). Analysis is invaluable when you have the time to research and plan evidence-based care but if you rely too much on analysis, you are likely to ignore important sensory or emotional information cues (e.g. Nigel focused on the absence of a cotton bud and did not notice the inflammation or acknowledge that Angela had a problem; he was also unaware of how his verbal and non-verbal communication made things worse).

Clinical decision-making in nursing and healthcare can often make the difference between a person surviving or dying from an illness or injury. So, it is vital that clinical judgement and decision-making is accurate in diagnosing problems and delivering safe and effective care. However, the case study showed that it is not an exact science and human error can lead to important information (e.g. signs and symptoms of ill health) being missed or misinterpreted. This is why it makes sense to research clinical decision-making in order to learn more about it, develop better skills and competence, and reduce the likelihood of errors and mistakes.

Each of the nine modes of practice has strengths and weaknesses and the idea is to use the most appropriate one to match the nature of the problem you are about to tackle. To be able to do this you need to develop knowledge and skills in all nine modes of practice. The next section will develop your understanding a bit more by asking you to apply the nine modes of practice to a case study regarding a nursing student's experience of patient assessment.

Applying nine modes of practice to a nursing student's patient assessment

As a student nurse you can rightly expect to receive guidance and role modelling in decision-making from registered nurses, mentors and other health professionals. However, unless you go about in a permanent trance you are making decisions independently every moment of your waking life, including during practice placements, as the following case study shows.

> **Case study: Assessing Vicky's complaint of being 'stressed out' and deciding what to do**
>
> *Marion is a second-year nursing student doing a community placement. It includes working with a school nurse who looks after pupils' health needs (e.g. first aid, health education, support, advice, immunisation checks) at a large comprehensive school. Vicky, age 14, goes to the school nurse's office and asks Marion if she can give her something for her 'nerves'. Marion explains that she is not the nurse, who should be back in 20 minutes, and asks Vicky if she wants to wait or come back. Vicky opts to stay and tells Marion that she hates coming to school and that it's 'stressing her out'. Marion asks if there is anything in particular that she finds stressful about school. Vicky describes feeling frightened and embarrassed because Sue, an older pupil, 'has a crush' on her, keeps trying to kiss her on the lips, follows her around both at school and on the way home, and will not stop stalking her despite Vicky saying, 'Stay away from me'. When Vicky rejected her advances Sue apparently got angry and told her parents that a head wound she received (during a fight with a young woman who kicked her when she was lying on the floor) was caused by Vicky attacking her. Sue's parents then accosted Vicky and her mum in their car outside an ice-skating club (where they knew Vicky went), verbally abused them, kicked the car, broke a door mirror and punched Vicky's mum when she told them to stop. Vicky says she cannot sleep, is 'off her food', feels sick all the time, is really scared of Sue and wants Marion to give her something that will 'make it all go away'.*
>
> *While Vicky is telling her shocking story, Marion wonders what she has let herself in for as she feels completely out of her depth. Just then she remembers a lecture on safeguarding vulnerable people and she realises that she is duty-bound to tell the school nurse what Vicky has said. The school nurse returns to the office and Marion briefs her about how she has handled Vicky's request for help, and the gist of her problems. The school nurse says Marion has done well to enable Vicky to talk and it is important to keep a record of this and report the matter to the head teacher, Vicky's teacher, parents and GP after she has spoken to Vicky.*

Vicky's case study shows that you never quite know what might happen during your clinical placements. When something unexpected does happen you often have to think on your feet and make a decision on the spot without the benefit of advice from a senior colleague or the opportunity to research how you should respond. Activity 10.3 asks you to review Marion's decision-making in caring for Vicky with reference to Standing's nine modes of practice.

Activity 10.3 — Critical thinking and decision-making

> The purpose of this activity is to give you some practice in applying decision theory to patient assessment and decision-making. Look back at how the nine modes of practice were used to review decision-making in Angela's case study, and then try to apply as many of the nine modes you think are appropriate to the decision-making evident in Vicky's case study.

Chapter 10

continued ...

Nine modes of practice	Examples of decision-making in Vicky's case study
Intuitive judgement	
Reflective judgement	
Patient and peer-aided judgement	
System-aided judgement	
Critical review of experiential and research evidence	
Action research and clinical audit	
Qualitative research	
Survey research	
Experimental research	

An outline answer is given at the end of the chapter.

A matrix model of nursing students' perceptions of clinical decision-making

Both Angela's and Vicky's case studies provide a glimpse of what it is like to be a student nurse (Kim and Marion) during practice placements, observing, reflecting on experience and developing skills in patient assessment, clinical judgement and decision-making. A research study of nursing students' reflections on developing decision-making skills created a matrix model that describes ten perceptions (key aspects) of clinical decision-making (Standing, 2014). Table 10.3 lists the ten perceptions of decision-making identified by the nursing students in Standing's research study together with a brief description of each one.

Collaborative	Consulting with patients, relatives, nurses, mentors and health professionals to inform relevant patient-centred decisions
Observation	Use of senses to assess patients' physical and mental health, monitor vital signs, review investigations, record responses to nursing/healthcare interventions and report any concerns
Systematic	Using critical thinking and problem-solving skills to assess problems, set goals, deliver care and evaluate outcomes
Standardised	Application of NHS trust policies, procedures and care plans, research evidence-based clinical guidelines and assessment tools

Prioritising	Risk assessment and management to avoid causing harm to any patient, targeting care on those with more serious problems first, and safeguarding the vulnerable, e.g. physical/mental disability
Experience and intuition	Recognising similarities and differences in current and previous situations, being guided by what worked before, not repeating mistakes, realising you may lack the experience to make a decision
Reflective	Reviewing events as they happen (reflection in action) or looking back (reflection on action) for insight into the best course of action
Ethical sensitivity	Applying ethical principles (autonomy, justice, beneficence, non-maleficence) to ensure patients' human rights are respected, e.g. maintaining confidentiality, gaining informed consent to procedures
Accountability	Being answerable to patients, public, NHS trusts, Nursing and Midwifery Council and the legal system for the consequences of your actions and being able to explain, justify and defend your decisions when asked to do so
Confidence	Self-assurance from experience and achievements and professional assurance that give patients and colleagues confidence in you

Table 10.3: Matrix model – ten perceptions of clinical decision-making in nursing

Activity 10.4 — Reflection

Take a moment to think about the matrix model – the ten perceptions of clinical decision-making in nursing. Remember that this description of clinical decision-making came from pooling nursing students' reflections of their experiences in clinical practice. Does it tally with your experience? Can you relate to the different aspects of decision-making that are identified? Can you think of any other aspects that are not incorporated in the matrix model? How do you think it compares to the cognitive continuum theory – the nine modes of practice?

As this is for your own reflection, no outline answer is provided.

Comparing the nine modes of practice and ten perceptions of clinical decision-making

The ten perceptions of decision-making, like the nine modes of practice, is an evidence-based tool to guide and evaluate patient assessment, clinical judgement and decision-making. Both describe a range of knowledge and skills and there are some clear similarities between them, as shown below.

Similarities in some of the modes of practice and perceptions of clinical decision-making

Modes of practice	Perceptions of clinical decision-making
Intuitive judgement	Experience and intuition
Reflective judgement	Reflective
Patient and peer-aided judgement	Collaborative
System-aided judgement	Systematic
Action research and clinical audit	Standardised

Due to their similarity, applying the above modes of practice and perceptions of decision-making to guide or review patient assessment would more or less cover the same ground. For example, if, when doing Activity 10.3, you interpreted Marion's rapport with Vicky as an example of 'patient and peer-aided judgement', it would also be an example of 'collaborative' clinical decision-making if you were applying the matrix model. However, the other four modes of practice are more clearly research-focused (critical review of experiential and research evidence, qualitative, survey and experimental research). In contrast, the other five perceptions of decision-making are more clearly clinically focused (observation, prioritising, ethical sensitivity, accountability and confidence). To get an idea of what these perceptions of decision-making have to offer it is worth seeing what light they cast on Vicky's case study (see Table 10.4).

Perceptions of clinical decision-making	Examples of decision-making in Vicky's case study
Observation	Marion observed that Vicky wanted something to make the stress go away; that she was prepared to wait to see the school nurse; that she was responsive to Marion asking probing questions about what might have led to her feeling stressed at school; and that, given her account of events, it was understandable that she should feel stressed out.
Prioritising	Marion and the school nurse identified that taking steps to protect Vicky from abuse and to ensure her safety was the main priority.
Ethical sensitivity	Marion respected Vicky's autonomy in choosing to tell someone about her problem; she was aware of the sensitive and confidential nature of their discussion while realising she had a duty to report it to the appropriate authorities; her actions appeared to help Vicky (beneficence) explain what was upsetting her, and help protect her from bullying, harassment and intimidation (maleficence) by Sue in the foreseeable future.

Accountability	Marion and the school nurse realised that the school has a duty to provide a safe environment for pupils and to take action where risks are identified; they also had to document what had happened as they might be called upon to explain and justify their actions.
Confidence	Marion's confidence was initially shaken when she found out the seriousness of Vicky's problems; she recovered her composure by focusing on safeguarding Vicky against further potential abuse; and her confidence was boosted when the school nurse said she did well.

Table 10.4: Perceptions of clinical decision-making applied to Vicky's case study

Activity 10.5 — Critical thinking and decision-making

Take a moment to look back at Activity 10.3, where you applied the nine modes of practice to review patient assessment in Vicky's case study. Now look at the above application of five perceptions of decision-making and reflect on whether they help to identify any aspects of patient assessment that you did not find out using the nine modes of practice.

As this is for your own reflection, no outline answer is provided.

Both cognitive continuum theory and the matrix model offer evidence-based frameworks to guide, review and develop clinical judgement and decision-making in patient assessment. The matrix model is particularly relevant in pre-registration nurse education as the ten perceptions of decision-making come from nursing students' reflections on their clinical experiences. It also complements previous chapters by encouraging a co-operative, person-centred, holistic (bio-psycho-social-spiritual), ethical and health-promoting approach to patient assessment.

Applying the matrix model to patient assessment, clinical decision-making and healthcare

Successfully delivering person-centred/holistic patient assessment, clinical decision-making and healthcare sounds lovely in theory but making it happen in reality is very challenging. As health professionals become more technically skilled, their clinical focus tends to narrow on specific aspects of care and this can go against seeing patients as unique individuals. The next case study shows the problems that can occur when this happens.

Chapter 10

Case study: A lesson in patient assessment and holistic care from Francis and his family

Francis, age 39, has received mental health care for 20 years since he was diagnosed as suffering from paranoid schizophrenia during his first year at university. When Francis is well, he is a shy, artistic, thoughtful and placid person. When unwell he is convinced that people want to harm him (when they don't), and these false beliefs (delusions of persecution) are resistant to reason or evidence that challenges them. He may also hear voices (auditory hallucinations), which can make him agitated and aggressive. Francis's mental health has been stabilised through medication (e.g. clozapine, an antipsychotic drug) and support from his family and community agencies. His mum, Elizabeth, and dad, Jeffrey, live in the same town and encourage Francis to visit or stay with them whenever he wishes. The parents never go away on holiday together to make sure that one of them is always available if he needs them. He has a younger brother, James, living 60 miles away, who he likes to talk to on the phone.

Two months ago Francis found that he could not move his left arm or feel his fingers so he went to the GP surgery. He saw a GP who did not detect that anything was wrong. A few days later Jeffrey saw Francis and was worried about his inability to move his left arm. Jeffrey took Francis to an out-of-hours service at a local NHS trust hospital where the duty GP said Francis might benefit from physiotherapy but no referral was made. A week later there was no change. Elizabeth was so concerned that she took Francis to see the GP and insisted that something was done to find out why he could not move his left arm. The GP referred Francis to have a computed tomography (CT) scan to check for problems.

On the day of the scan, Elizabeth asked Francis to take a lorazepam tablet (as prescribed) to reduce his anxiety, she accompanied him to the hospital and the CT scan was carried out. They were not told the result, but a week later Francis got a letter with an urgent appointment for a magnetic resonance imaging (MRI) scan. No reason was given, and this made Francis very anxious.

Elizabeth went to see the GP to ask for an explanation and was told the CT scan showed an abnormality in Francis's brain that needed further investigation. She prepared and accompanied Francis for the MRI scan (as she had done for the CT scan) and it was carried out without incident. They were not told the result, but a week later Francis got a telephone call from the GP, asking him to pick up a referral letter from the surgery and take it to the emergency care unit of the local hospital for him to be admitted.

Francis was upset and anxious and he called his mother. Elizabeth was surprised the GP did not let her know about this so that she might support Francis. She took him to the emergency care unit, where a consultant informed them that the MRI scan indicated Francis had had a stroke (also called a cerebrovascular accident) due to haemorrhaging (bleeding) in his brain. Francis was transferred to a ward that assessed and treated patients with strokes.

Francis was admitted to the stroke ward by Julie, a third-year nursing student. The ward used an integrated care pathway to guide and co-ordinate the multidisciplinary healthcare team in key aspects of assessment and treatment of patients who had suffered from a stroke. Julie's initial assessment of Francis focused on identifying any impairment of sensation and movement in Francis's limbs, particularly in his left arm, and how long this had been so. She did not ask about Francis's previous medical history. Julie informed Francis that he would need to have another MRI scan, 'probably some time tomorrow'.

The next day Francis was getting increasingly anxious and distressed. He knew Elizabeth was at work so he phoned his brother James and began crying, saying, 'I don't know what is going on'. James assured Francis that he would drive down to see him in the afternoon. In the meantime a hospital porter asked Francis to sit in a wheelchair and took him to have his second MRI scan. The nurses were busy at the time and no one explained to Francis where he was being taken. At the MRI unit Francis was highly anxious, very distressed and agitated. He started swearing and screaming at the staff not to touch him when they tried to do the MRI scan.

Francis was taken back to the ward. When James arrived he was still agitated and bad-tempered, shouting and swearing at the nurses who were unsure how to deal with him. He complained of pain in his left arm, which was bruised from unsuccessful attempts to insert an intravenous line in the MRI unit. James tried to calm Francis down but he was too upset and so James called their mother. Elizabeth came straight away and she managed to comfort Francis and get him to relax a little bit, assuring him that nobody there really wanted to hurt him. The next day Elizabeth got the consultant to agree to discharge Francis to the care of his family who would prepare and accompany him for further tests or treatments as an outpatient.

Francis's case study provides a graphic account of how important accurate patient assessment is and how difficult it can sometimes be for doctors and nurses to achieve this. When things do not go as well as they should, it is vital to learn from the experience in order to improve. Francis and his family demonstrated many of the skills in person-centred, holistic patient assessment and care that nurses and other health professionals can learn from, as shown in Table 10.5.

Collaborative	Francis informed the GP about his arm problem; Jeffrey took Francis for a second opinion from a GP at the out-of-hours service; James came to support Francis when he was distressed
Observation	Francis and his parents saw that he had lost the ability to move his left arm, recognised that it needed investigation and alerted the GP
Systematic	Elizabeth carefully prepared Francis for the CT and MRI scans by explaining what they were for, accompanying him to the hospital and supporting him during procedures to help relieve his anxiety
Standardised	Francis continued taking prescribed antipsychotic medication; Elizabeth also asked him to take prescribed lorazepam tablets on the day of the scan to help control and relieve his anxiety
Prioritising	When Francis's weakness in his left arm did not improve, Elizabeth insisted that the GP arrange for the problem to be investigated
Experience and intuition	Francis and his family sensed that something was physically wrong with him despite not knowing that he had had a stroke at that time
Reflective	Francis's family were aware of his mental fragility if stressed and realised that they had to support and nurse him through the investigations and procedures to avoid him becoming disturbed

Ethical sensitivity	Francis's family respected his autonomy – when he said something was wrong with his arm they believed him (and were right to); and they applied beneficence by being very caring toward him
Accountability	Francis's family took responsibility for arranging for his discharge from hospital because the poor care he received was upsetting him; they looked after him at home while supporting him during further investigations and treatment for the stroke as an outpatient
Confidence	Francis had confidence in his family's ability to help him because they saw beyond his diagnosis of paranoid schizophrenia and knew him as a unique person whom they loved and cared for. His family knew that while he was taking antipsychotic medication Francis was receptive to their attempts to explain things and help him

Table 10.5: Ten perceptions of clinical decision-making applied by Francis and family

Francis's case study reveals the challenges in applying the theory of person-centred, holistic assessment and care to practice. Francis's medical history of long-term mental illness appears to have got in the way of doctors and nurses being attentive to his physical and psychological needs. This is evident in the initial failure to take his physical complaint about not being able to move his arm seriously. Once it was clear that Francis had suffered a stroke, he was not given the care and psychological support in hospital that anyone would be entitled to receive. Francis and his family demonstrated how he should have been cared for by the doctors and nurses. This emphasises the importance of being open-minded, carefully observing patients, communicating with them and taking note of what they say to ensure that assessment and related care decisions are relevant to their specific individual needs. Applying the matrix model to patient assessment, decision-making and care interventions can help nurses to succeed in relating theory in person-centred, holistic care to the reality of clinical practice.

Applying a 'PERSON' evaluation tool to review and enhance patient assessment and decision-making in nursing

So far in this chapter we have looked at the interrelationship between patient assessment, clinical judgement and decision-making and related nursing interventions. We also applied relevant theory and research findings to help identify, develop, understand and apply a range of key knowledge, skills and attitudes to patient assessment. As the above case study shows, healthcare professionals can make mistakes and patients suffer as a result. We therefore need to continually evaluate patient assessment, care plans and decision-making to identify where we can improve. Evaluating nursing decisions in assessing, planning and delivering patient care has been defined as follows:

A critical review of nursing decisions and associated care in: (i) addressing patients' rights, needs, problems and preferences; (ii) avoiding causing harm to patients; (iii) carrying out interventions that have beneficial outcomes for patients; (iv) applying relevant evidence, research and clinical guidelines to patient care; (v) identifying strengths and weaknesses of care provided; and (vi) considering the implications of the findings for continuing patient care and our own professional development and education needs as nurses.
(Standing, 2014, p201)

This definition of what evaluating nursing decisions means was developed in response to the publication of the Francis Report (2013). The Francis Report highlighted unacceptable standards of care in an NHS trust whose priority was meeting certain health targets (e.g. quantity of patients processed) rather than quality of care patients received. Patients and relatives concerns and complaints were ignored; unsafe, ineffective care with poor patient outcomes was allowed to continue for years; and healthcare professionals were discouraged from 'whistle blowing' about this. Evaluating nursing decisions must therefore focus on patients' experiences and feedback about care they receive, identify better ways of delivering safe and effective care addressing their needs and health problems, and prompt nurses to be open and honest in reviewing their actions and be committed to developing their clinical competence. A 'PERSON' evaluation tool was developed to address all of the points in the above definition and this can be applied within any of the nursing pathways (Adult, Child, Mental Health, Learning Disability). It also summarises professional standards of conduct which nurses must adhere to (NMC, 2008, 2015). The 'PERSON' acronym stands for the following:

P = Patient-centred

E = Evidence-based

R = Risks assessed and managed

S = Safe and effective delivery of care

O = Outcomes of care benefit the patient

N = Nursing and midwifery strengths and weaknesses

In order to evaluate nursing decisions using each element of the 'PERSON' evaluation tool a series of questions was devised for nurses to answer in reviewing the quality of care they have provided, as described in Table 10.6.

'PERSON' acronym	Answer questions to evaluate decisions
Patient-centred	Were different care options explained to the patient?
	Did the patient give consent before the intervention?
	How did the patient's opinion contribute to care plans?
	If for any reason the patient was unable to contribute to decisions, how were his or her rights safeguarded?
Evidence-based	What patient observations indicated a need for action?
	What corroborating evidence supports your assessment?
	What was the rationale for the selected intervention?
	What research evidence underpins the intervention?

Chapter 10

(Continued)

'PERSON' acronym	Answer questions to evaluate decisions
Risks assessed and managed	What threats to patient's health/wellbeing were there?
	What was done to ensure a safe healthcare environment?
	What procedure did you follow to control known risks?
	How did you escalate concerns if problems worsened?
Safe and effective delivery of care	What knowledge/skills/attitudes were applied to care?
	What prior experience did you have of this intervention?
	How was your competence to give care quality assured?
	How did you share information on the care you gave?
Outcomes of care benefit the patient	What was the patient's/relatives' feedback about care?
	To what extent were desired outcomes of care achieved?
	How do you think the patient benefitted from this care?
	How will you address any negative outcomes of care?
Nursing and midwifery strengths and weaknesses	What did you learn from this experience of patient care?
	How did you justify public trust in your ability to care?
	On reflection, what could you have done differently?
	What are you doing to improve decision-making skills?

Table 10.6: Clinical decision-making 'PERSON' evaluation tool (Standing, 2014, p204)

The 'PERSON' evaluation tool also incorporates relevant decision theory (nine modes of practice) and research (ten perceptions of clinical decision-making) discussed earlier in the chapter. For example, there is a strong emphasis on nurses respecting patients' human rights, collaborating with patients, colleagues and others, using observation and prioritising skills, and being systematic, reflective and accountable in delivering and critically reviewing patient care. Table 10.7 applies the 'PERSON' evaluation tool to review Marion's assessment of Vicky in the second case study.

PATIENT-CENTRED

Were different care options explained to the patient? Marion gave Vicky the option of waiting or coming back in 20 minutes when the registered school nurse would be there.

Did the patient give consent before the intervention? Vicky chose to wait and voluntarily began telling Marion about her problems.

How did the patient's opinion contribute to care plans? Vicky wanted something to be done to help her deal with feeling 'stressed out'.

If for any reason the patient was unable to contribute to decisions, how were his or her rights safeguarded? Vicky is a vulnerable minor who reported being abused. To safeguard her, subsequent decisions would need to involve her parents, teachers and GP.

EVIDENCE-BASED

What patient observations indicated a need for action? Vicky went to the school nurse's office seeking help, was not put off when she wasn't there, and she described physical and psychological symptoms associated with anxiety and stress in relation to her account of being intimidated and assaulted by Sue.

What corroborating evidence supports your assessment? Marion only had Vicky's account of events to go on at the time but it did explain why she felt 'stressed out' and why she wanted help to deal with it.

What was the rationale for the selected intervention? Marion applied listening, communication and interpersonal skills in responding to Vicky's wish to talk about her problems, and enabling her to do so.

What research evidence underpins the intervention? The skills Marion applied are underpinned by principles of therapeutic communication derived from humanistic psychology (Bach and Grant, 2011). In researching what nursing students associated with being a nurse, their conceptions of nursing included 'Listening and being there', 'communicating', and 'empathising and non-judgemental' (Standing, 2014).

RISKS ASSESSED AND MANAGED

What threats to patient's health/wellbeing were there? Vicky's physical health was a concern as she indicated she was not eating properly/felt sick, and said she had been verbally and physically assaulted. Her mental health was also a concern as she was frightened, anxious, and felt unable to cope.

What was done to ensure a safe healthcare environment? The school nurse's office provided a place of safety for pupils to discuss personal and confidential issues affecting their health and wellbeing.

What procedure did you follow to control known risks? Marion made it clear to Vicky that she was not the school nurse, but that she would be back in 20 minutes. In this way she acknowledged her limitations in competence (NMC, 2008, 2015), and that the school nurse was supervising her clinical placement.

How did you escalate concerns if problems worsened? When it became clear that Vicky's problems were of a serious nature affecting her health and wellbeing both in and outside school Marion realised that she was unable to resolve these issues herself and she had a duty to report this to the school nurse.

SAFE AND EFFECTIVE DELIVERY OF CARE

What knowledge/skills/attitudes were applied to care? In addition to the communication skills discussed above Marion remembered a lecture regarding safeguarding and this helped her to understand that Vicky is a vulnerable minor who needs to be protected from harm.

What prior experience did you have of this intervention? Marion had no experience of dealing with this challenging situation.

How was your competence to give care quality assured? Marion recognised that she was out of her depth given the seriousness of Vicky's problems and that the school nurse needed to deal with it.

How did you share information on the care you gave? Marion informed the school nurse about how she had responded to Vicky's request for help and all the details of the problems that she described. The school nurse also asked Marion to write notes on what Vicky had told her as a formal record.

(Continued)

> **OUTCOMES OF CARE BENEFIT THE PATIENT**
>
> **What was the patient's/relatives' feedback about care?** The case study does not give details of Vicky's response to Marion's care. Her willingness to talk to Marion suggests that she felt comfortable doing so.
>
> **To what extent were desired outcomes of care achieved?** Vicky wanted Marion to give her something to make the stress go away suggesting that she was looking for medication to relieve anxiety which Marion was not in a position to give. However, Marion's interventions helped to uncover the causes of Vicky's fear and anxiety which laid the foundation for the alleged bullying and intimidation to be dealt with.
>
> **How do you think the patient benefitted from this care?** It took a lot of courage for Vicky to confide in someone about her problems and if Marion had not been welcoming and approachable Vicky might have gone away, not come back, had her sense of being victimised reinforced, and her problems unresolved.
>
> **How will you address any negative outcomes of care?** While Marion coped well with the situation, being left on her own to deal with pupils' health problems poses risks which needs to be managed more effectively in future. For example, not being left alone or calling the school nurse to supervise/deal with problems.
>
> **NURSING AND MIDWIFERY STRENGTHS AND WEAKNESSES**
>
> **What did you learn from this experience of patient care?** Marion gained valuable experience in communicating with Vicky to assess why she was feeling 'stressed out'. She was also able to apply the theory of safeguarding to clinical practice which reinforced her understanding. The school nurse said that she had done well and this helped to validate Marion's positive learning experience.
>
> **How did you justify public trust in your ability to care?** Marion put her feelings of being shocked by what Vicky told her to one side in order to behave in a professional manner. She focused on what Vicky needed from her and recognised that she needed to tell the school nurse about this situation.
>
> **On reflection, what could you have done differently?** The school nurse told Marion she needed to produce a written report of her interactions with Vicky. With hindsight it would be helpful for Marion to get in the habit of making notes or filling in forms during assessments. This would help to structure interviews, ensure vital details are included, reduce recall errors, and aide accurate documentation.
>
> **What are you doing to improve decision-making skills?** Marion is a second-year student so she will continue to learn about decision-making skills during her nursing degree. She will also reflect on this episode of care and may incorporate this in her personal and professional development portfolio.

Table 10.7: Applying the 'PERSON' evaluation tool to review Marion's assessment of Vicky

The above example shows how applying the 'PERSON' evaluation tool offers a comprehensive framework to evaluate nursing decisions. It does so by incorporating relevant decision theory and research, nurses' professional code of conduct, and the recommendations of the Francis Report. It is a person-centred system quality assuring safe and effective nursing care which requires nurses to be honest to acknowledge errors and their development needs. In this way it also addresses current health policy priorities (DH, 2012) by promoting the '6Cs' of compassionate care (care, compassion, competence, communication, courage, commitment). It is recommended that you use this tool to guide and evaluate your decision-making, and to structure your personal and professional development portfolios.

Chapter summary

This chapter has shown you how assessing health problems involves clinical judgement (intuition, reflection, critical thinking) in reaching a diagnosis and considering possible courses of action. Clinical decision-making is where a choice is made about which care intervention to use. Two frameworks (cognitive continuum theory – nine modes of practice – and matrix model – ten perceptions of clinical decision-making) were offered to guide the development, application and review of clinical judgement and decision-making skills. A 'PERSON' evaluation tool to guide and evaluate assessment, care plans and nursing interventions was then discussed. The 'PERSON' evaluation tool is recommended for you to use as it incorporates relevant decision theory and research, NMC standards of conduct, current health policy priorities, and addresses the Francis Report recommendations. It also complements person-centred, holistic patient assessment, care planning and nursing interventions which are advocated throughout this book.

Activities: brief outline answers

Activity 10.1 Reflection [page 140]

You may have included some of the following points:

Person doing assessment	Problems they identified	Their decision-making/action
Angela	Cotton bud stuck in left ear, pain, discomfort, dizziness, cannot concentrate on work, unable to bear it anymore	Try unsuccessfully to remove cotton bud, take paracetamol tablets to relieve pain, ask GP and nurses to remove it
First GP	Foreign body in left ear, pain and discomfort reported by Angela	Try unsuccessfully to remove it, refer to practice nurse for ear irrigation to remove it
Practice nurse	Foreign body in left ear, as advised by GP	Unable to do ear irrigation (equipment not working), refer Angela to the MIU

(Continued)

Person doing assessment	Problems they identified	Their decision-making/action
Nigel (nurse practitioner)	No foreign body in left ear, no health problem evident	Request second opinion from nurse practitioner colleague, refuse to do ear irrigation, discharge Angela from MIU
Helen (nurse practitioner)	No foreign body in left ear	Attend to another patient
Kim (student nurse)	Angela was getting irritated, sensed that she was not well	Keep quiet and just observe, reflecting on feeling torn between respect for Nigel and empathising with Angela
Second GP	No foreign body in left ear, left ear inflamed and infected	Prescribe antibiotics (by mouth), refer to ENT
ENT consultant	No foreign body in left ear, left ear still appears infected	Prescribe antibiotic ear drops, confirm ear irrigation not appropriate, give health promotion advice to Angela, i.e. stop putting cotton buds in ears, use ear drops instead

Activity 10.3 Critical thinking and decision-making [page 145]

You may have included some of the following points:

Nine modes of practice	Examples of decision-making in Vicky's case study
Intuitive judgement	Vicky felt unable to cope so she sought help; Marion sensed that Vicky needed to talk to someone; Marion felt 'completely out of her depth' at one point.
Reflective judgement	Just when Marion was thinking she did not know what she was doing, she remembered a safeguarding lecture, and realised she had a duty to report Vicky's problems to an appropriate authority (given that Vicky is a vulnerable minor, aged 14, who has reported being abused).
Patient and peer-aided judgement	Marion did not send Vicky away (after she had got up the courage to speak to someone about her problem) and she enabled Vicky to tell her what was 'stressing her out'; Marion reported the matter to the school nurse which influenced her subsequent action (e.g. inform head teacher, explore issues further with Vicky).

System-aided judgement	The school nursing service is part of the organisational judgement structure of the school and pupils know they can seek help there for health-related problems; Marion and the school nurse appeared to understand that they had a moral and legal duty to report Vicky's suspected abuse.
Critical review of experiential and research evidence	The school nurse gave Marion positive feedback for her role in enabling Vicky to talk about her problems.
Action research and clinical audit	The school nurse was aware that formal records needed to be kept of what Vicky had said which may be subject to official scrutiny; the school nurse recognised that Vicky's suspected abuse requires further action to be taken by the head teacher, Vicky's teacher, parents and GP to ensure Vicky's safety at (and to and from) school.
Qualitative research	Vicky's experience of care by the school nursing service is a qualitative case study.
Survey research	A database records allegations/instances of abuse of vulnerable children by schools and social services.
Experimental research	Although unrelated to Vicky's problem, immunisation programmes (with which school nurses may be involved) are developed and tested through scientific research.

Further reading

Standing, M (2014) *Clinical Judgement and Decision-Making for Nursing Students.* London: SAGE Publications.

In-depth application of the matrix model (a chapter is devoted to each of the ten perceptions of clinical decision-making in nursing) demonstrated using case studies. Plus a more detailed account of the 'PERSON' evaluation tool.

Useful website

www.nice.org.uk

National Institute for Health and Care Excellence website, where you can find a wide variety of evidence-based assessment tools and clinical guidelines.

Glossary

Anaemia: lack of haemoglobin which lowers the oxygen carrying capacity of the red blood cells.

Arteriogram: injection of substance which shows up on X-ray to outline arterial vessels.

Body language: body movements and expressions which reveal emotions.

Clinical decision-making: applies clinical judgement to select the best possible evidence-based option to control risks and address patients' needs in high quality care for which you are accountable.

Clinical judgement: informed opinion (using intuition, reflection and critical thinking) that relates observation and assessment of patients to identifying and evaluating alternative nursing options.

Cognitive continuum: judgement ranging from intuitive hunches to critical analysis which is tailored to the constantly changing nature of clinical demands and health problems we deal with.

Cruse: bereavement support service.

CVA (cerebrovascular accident): also known as a stroke, this is an interruption to blood flow in a vessel in the brain due to either a clot or rupture.

Delirious: suffering from confusion caused by fever.

ECG (electrocardiogram): a procedure which records the electrical activity of the heart and produces a tracing of this.

Epigastric pain: pain in the upper abdominal region.

Exudate: leakage from a wound.

Fibroadenoma: a collection of fibrous and glandular cells which form a mobile lump with distinct boundaries.

Glasgow Coma Scale: this is a neurological scale that measures levels of consciousness.

Glucocorticoid: a group of hormones released by the adrenal cortex.

Hypoglycaemia: low blood sugar level.

Idiocultures: the knowledge systems and ways of behaving of a small group of people.

Ingest: eat or drink.

Mindfulness: focusing on and becoming acutely aware of things normally taken for granted.

Neurological: arising from the nervous system.

Neuropathy: loss of peripheral sensation particularly in the feet due to damaged nerve endings and reduced blood flow.

Oesophageal gastroduodenoscopy: a procedure in which a flexible tube with a camera is passed through the oesophagus, stomach and duodenum to visualise the internal lining and structure.

'PERSON' evaluation tool: A new universal framework to question, evaluate and guide nursing and midwifery decisions/interventions in the six key areas, namely: **P**atient-centred/**E**vidence-based/**R**isks assessed and managed/**S**afe and effective delivery of care/**O**utcomes benefit the patient/**N**ursing and midwifery strengths and weaknesses.

Prognosis: predicted course of the disease.

Stent: a corrugated metal or plastic cylindrical tube inserted into a vessel to maintain its patency.

Ulcerative colitis: inflammatory disease of the large bowel.

Urisheath: a device which covers the penis directing urine into a tube which empties into a bag.

References

Aggleton, P and Chalmers, H (2000) *Nursing Models and Nursing Practice*, 2nd edn. Basingstoke: Palgrave.

Andrews, J and Butler, M (2014) *Trusted to Care*. Available at: http://wales.gov.uk/docs/dhss/publications/140512trustedtocareen.pdf

Anthony, P and Crawford, P (2000) Service user involvement in care planning: the mental health nurse's perspective. *Journal of Psychiatric and Mental Health Nursing*, 7: 425–34.

Aschengrau, A and Seage, G (2013) *Essential Epidemiology in Public Health*, 3rd edn. Burlington, MA: Jones and Bartlett.

Aston, L, Wakefield, J and McGown, R (2010) *The Student Nurse Guide to Decision-Making in Practice*. Maidenhead: Open University Press.

Bach, S and Grant, A (2015) *Communication and Interpersonal Skills for Nurses*, 3rd edn. London: SAGE/Learning Matters.

Barker, J (2013) *Evidence-Based Practice for Nurses*, 2nd edn. London: SAGE Publications.

Barrett, D, Wilson, B and Woollands, A (2009) *Care Planning: A Guide for Nurses*. Harlow: Pearson Education.

Barrett, D, Wilson, B and Woollands, A (2012) *Care Planning: A Guide for Nurses*, 2nd edn. Harlow: Pearson Education.

Carnerio, I and Howard, N (2011) *Introduction to Epidemiology*, 2nd edn. Maidenhead: McGraw Open University Press.

Carpenito-Moyet, LJ (2013) *Handbook of Nursing Diagnosis*, 14th edn. Philadelphia: Wolters Kluwer Health/Lippincott Williams Wilkins.

Carper, B (1978) Fundamental patterns of knowing in nursing. *Advances in Nursing Science*, 1: 13–23.

Chapman, S (2010) Managing pain in the older person. *Nursing Standard*, 25: 35–9.

Clarke, J (2013) *Spiritual Care in Everyday Nursing Practice: A New Approach*. Basingstoke: Palgrave Macmillan.

Defloor, T, Clark, M, Witherow, A et al. (2005) EPAUP statement on prevalence and incidence monitoring of pressure ulcer occurrence 2005. *European Pressure Ulcer Advisory Panel*, 6: 69–85.

Department of Health (2000) *The NHS Plan*. London: The Stationery Office.

Department of Health (2006) *Your Health, Your Care, Your Say*. London: The Stationery Office.

Department of Health (2009) *Long Term Conditions: Care Planning*. Available from: www.dh.gov.uk/en/Healthcare/Longtermconditions/DH_093359

Department of Health (2010) *Ready to Go? Planning the Discharge and the Transfer of Patients from Hospital and Intermediate Care*. London: The Stationery Office.

Department of Health and NHS Commissioning Board (2012) *Compassion in Practice: Nursing, Midwifery and Care Staff, Our Vision and Strategy*. Available from: www.england.nhs.uk/wp-content/uploads/2012/12/compassion-in-practice.pdf

Dewing, J (2004) Concerns relating to the application of frameworks to promote person-centredness in nursing with older people. *Journal of Clinical Nursing*, 13: 39–44.

Dewing, J (2008) Personhood and dementia: revisiting Tom Kitwood's ideas. *International Journal of Older People Nursing*, 3: 3–13.

Dougherty, L and Lister, S (eds) (2011) *The Royal Marsden Hospital Manual of Clinical Nursing Procedures*, student edition, 8th edn. Oxford: Wiley-Blackwell.

Dyson, S (2004) Transcultural nursing care of adults. In Husband, C and Terry, B (eds) *Transcultural Health Care Practice: An Educational Resource for Nurses and Health Care Practitioners*. London: RCN.

Egan, G (2014) *The Skilled Helper: A Problem Management and Opportunity Development Approach to Helping*, 10th edn. Belmont, CA: Brooks/Cole.

Ellis, P (2013) *Evidence-Based Practice in Nursing*, 2nd edn. London: SAGE Publications.

Equality and Human Rights Commission (2011) Inquiry into home care of older people. Available from: www.equalityhumanrights.com/legal-and-policy/our-legal-work/inquiries-and-assessments/inquiry-into-home-care-of-older-people

Evans, DMD, Evans, C and Evans, RA (2003) *Special Tests: The Procedure and Meaning of Common Tests in Hospital*, 15th edn. Philadelphia, PA: Elsevier.

Field, L and Smith, B (2008) *Nursing Care: An Essential Guide*. Harlow: Pearson Education.

Figley, C (1995) Compassion fatigue: to a new understanding of the costs of caring. In Stamm, R and Hudnell, B (eds) *Secondary Traumatic Stress: Self Care Issues for Clinicians, Researchers and Educators*. Baltimore, MD: The Sidran Press, pp3–28.

Francis, R (2013) *Report of the Mid Staffordshire NHS Foundation Trust Public Inquiry: Executive Summary*. London: HMSO. Available from: www.midstaffspublicinquiry.com/sites/default/files/report/Executive%20summary.pdf.

Frosh, S (2002) *After Words: The Personal in Gender, Culture and Psychotherapy*. Basingstoke: Palgrave.

Funkesson, KH, Anbäcken, EM and Ek, AC (2007) Nurses' reasoning process during care planning taking pressure ulcer prevention as an example: a think aloud study. *International Journal of Nursing Studies*, 44: 1109–19.

Gillam, S, Yates, J and Badrinath, J (2007) *Essential Public Health*. Cambridge: Cambridge University Press.

Girard, NJ (2007) Do you know what you don't know? *AORN Journal*, 86: 177–8.

Goodman, B and Clemow, R (2010) *Nursing and Collaborative Practice*, 2nd edn. Exeter: Learning Matters.

Gordon, M (1994) *Nursing Diagnosis: Process and Application*. St Louis: Mosby Yearbook.

Hall, A (2005) Defining nursing knowledge. *Nursing Times*, 100: 34.

Hammond, KR (1996) *Human Judgement and Social Policy: Irreducible Uncertainty, Inevitable Error, Unavoidable Injustice*. New York: Oxford University Press.

Hawkey, B and Williams, J (2007) *The Role after Rehabilitation Nurse: RCN Guidance*. London: RCN.

Health Education England (2014) *NHS Five Year Forward View*. Available from: www.england.nhs.uk/wp-content/uploads/2014/10/5yfv-web.pdf

Hendrick, J (2000) *Law and Ethics in Nursing and Healthcare*. Cheltenham: Nelson Thornes.

Heron, J (1992) *Feeling and Personhood in Another Key*. London: SAGE.

Hillson, D and Murray-Webster, R (2007) *Understanding and Managing Risk Attitude*, 2nd edn. Farnham: Gower.

Hinchliff, S, Norman, S and Schober, J (eds) (2008) *Nursing Practice and Health Care*, 5th edn. London: Hodder Arnold.

Hogston, R and Marjoram, B (eds) (2011) *Foundations for Nursing Practice: Themes, Concepts and Frameworks*, 4th edn. Basingstoke: Palgrave Macmillan.

Holmes, S (2010) Importance of nutrition in palliative care of patients with chronic disease. *Nursing Standard*, 25: 48–56.

Howatson-Jones, L (2008) Outpatient nursing, in Howatson-Jones, L and Ellis, P (eds) *Outpatient, Day Surgery and Ambulatory Care*. Chichester: Wiley-Blackwell.

Howatson-Jones, L (2013) *Reflective Practice in Nursing*, 2nd edn. London: SAGE Publications.

Howatson-Jones, L and Ellis, P (eds) (2008) *Outpatient, Day Surgery and Ambulatory Care*. Chichester: Wiley-Blackwell.

Hutchfield, K (2010) *Information Skills for Nursing Students*. Exeter: Learning Matters.

Ikäheimo, H and Laitinen, A (2007) Dimensions of personhood. *Journal of Consciousness Studies*, 14 (5–6): 6–16.

Innes, A, Macpherson, S and McCabe, L (2006) *Promoting Person-Centred Care at the Frontline*. York: Joseph Rowntree Foundation.

Keogh, B (2013) Review into the quality of care and treatment provided by 14 hospital trusts in England: overview report. Available from: www.nhs.uk/NHSEngland/bruce-keogh-review/Documents/outcomes/keogh-review-final-report.pdf

References

Kitwood, T (1997) *Dementia Reconsidered: The Person Comes First*. Milton Keynes: Open University Press.

Lloyd, M (2010) *A Practical Guide to Care Planning in Health and Social Care*. Maidenhead: Open University Press.

Lynch, L, Hancox, K, Happell, B and Parker, J (2008) *Clinical Supervision for Nurses*. Chichester: Wiley-Blackwell.

Lyons, SS, Adams, S and Titler, M (2005) Falls prevention for older adults. *Journal of Gerontological Nursing*, 31: 9–14.

Malnutrition Advisory Group (2012) *Malnutrition Universal Screening Tool*. UK: Bapen. Available from: www.bapen.org.uk/screening-for-malnutrition/must/must-toolkit/the-must-itself

Manley K (2000) Organisational culture and consultant nurse outcomes: part 1 organisational culture. *Nursing Standard*, 14 (37): 34–8.

Manley, K and McCormack, B (2003) Practice development: purpose, methodology, facilitation and evaluation. *Nursing in Critical Care*, 8 (1): 22–9.

Manley, K, Sanders, K, Cardiff, S and Webster, J (2011) Effective workplace culture: the attributes, enabling factors and consequences of a new concept. *International Practice Development Journal*, 1 (2) Article 1. www.fons.org/library/journal/volume1-issue2/article1

McAllister, M (ed.) (2007) *Solution Focused Nursing*. Basingstoke: Palgrave.

McCabe, C and Timmins, F (2013) *Communication Skills for Nursing Practice*, 2nd edn. Basingstoke: Palgrave Macmillan.

McCormack, B (2004) Person-centredness in gerontological nursing: an overview of the literature. *Journal of Clinical Nursing*, 13: 31–8.

McCormack, B and McCance, T (2010) *The Theory and Practice of Person-Centredness in Nursing*. Oxford: Wiley-Blackwell.

McCormack, B, McCance, T and Maben, J (2013) Outcome evaluation in the development of person-centred practice. In McCormack, B, Manley, K and Titchen, A (eds) *Practice Development in Nursing and Healthcare*, 2nd edn. Chichester: Wiley-Blackwell, pp190–211.

Mental Capacity Act (2005) London: The Stationery Office.

Mental Health Act (1983) amended (2007) London: The Stationery Office.

Molly Case (2013) *Nursing the Nation*. Available from: www.youtube.com/watch?v=XOCda6OiYpg

Morris, RC (2012) The relative influence of values and identities on academic dishonesty: a quantitative analysis. *Current Research in Social Psychology*, 2: 1–20.

Moule, P and Goodman, M (2009) *Nursing Research: An Introduction*. London: SAGE Publications.

National Health Service (NHS) England (2014) *High Quality Care for All, Now and for Future Generations*. Available from: www.england.nhs.uk/ourwork/part-rel/transformation-fund/bcf-plan

National Institute for Health and Care Excellence (2005) *HNA: A Practical Guide*. London: National Institute for Health and Care Excellence.

National Institute for Health and Care Excellence (2006) *Nutrition Support for Adults, Oral Nutrition Support, Enteral Tube Feeding and Parental Nutrition*. Clinical guideline no. 32. London: National Collaborating Centre for Acute Care.

National Institute for Health and Care Excellence (2007) *Acutely Ill Patients in Hospital*. Clinical guideline no. 50. London: National Institute for Health and Care Excellence.

New South Wales Department of Health (2009) *Caring Together: The Health Action Plan for NSW, Sydney, NSW Department of Health*. New South Wales, Australia: Nursing and Midwifery Office, Essentials of Care Resource Guide Office of the NSW Department of Health. Last updated: 25 March 2011.

Nightingale, F (1860) *Notes on Nursing: What It Is and What It Is Not*. New York: Appleton.

Nolan, D and Ellis, P (2008) Communication and advocacy. In Howatson-Jones, L and Ellis, P (eds) *Outpatient, Day Surgery and Ambulatory Care*. Chichester: Wiley-Blackwell.

Northern Ireland Ombudsman (2013) Case Digest 25/11/13. Retrieved from: www.ni-ombudsman.org.uk/Publications.aspx

Nursing and Midwifery Council (2008) *The Code: Standards of Conduct, Performance and Ethics for Nurses and Midwives*. London: NMC.

Nursing and Midwifery Council (2010) *Guidance on Professional Conduct for Nursing and Midwifery Students*. London: NMC.

Nursing and Midwifery Council (2015) *The Code: Professional Standards of Practice and Behaviour for Nurses and Midwives*. London: NMC.

Orem, D (2001) *Nursing: Concepts of Practice*, 6th edn. London: Mosby.

Paans, W, Nieweg, RMB, van der Schans, CP et al. (2011) What factors influence the prevalence and accuracy of nursing diagnoses documentation in clinical practice? A systematic literature review. *Journal of Clinical Nursing*, 20: 2386–403.

Person-Centred Health and Care Collaborative (2014) *People at the Centre of Health and Care*. Available from: www.healthcareimprovementscotland.org/our_work/person-centred_care/person-centred_collaborative.aspx

Price, B (2002) Laddered questions and qualitative data research interviews. *Journal of Advanced Nursing*, 37: 273–81.

Pritchard, MJ (2009) Identifying and assessing anxiety in pre-operative patients. *Nursing Standard*, 23: 35–40.

Rogers, C (1995) *A Way of Being*. Boston, MA: Houghton Mifflin.

Roper, N, Logan, W and Tierney, A (2000) *The Roper–Logan–Tierney Model of Nursing: Based on Activities of Living*. Edinburgh: Churchill Livingstone.

Royal College of Nursing (2003) *Defining Nursing*. London: RCN.

Royal College of Nursing (2012) *Going Upstream: Nursing's Contribution to Public Health. Prevent, Promote and Protect*. London: RCN.

Royal College of Physicians (2012) *National Early Warning Score (NEWS): Standardising the Assessment of Acute-Illness Severity in the NHS. Report of a Working Party*. London: Royal College of Physicians. Available from: www.rcplondon.ac.uk/national-early-warning-score

Ruland, CM (1999) Decision support for patient preference-based care planning. *Journal of the American Medical Informatics Association*, 6: 304–12.

Rushforth, H (2009) *Assessment Made Incredibly Easy*. Philadelphia, PA: Lippincott, Williams and Wilkins.

Scottish Public Services Ombudsman (2014) Investigation reports. Available from: www.spso.org.uk/investigation-reports

Seedhouse, D (2009) *Ethics: The Heart of Healthcare*, 3rd edn. Chichester: John Wiley.

Sines, D, Saunders, M and Forbes-Burford, J (eds) (2009) *Community Health Care Nursing*, 4th edn. Chichester: Wiley Blackwell.

Standing, M (2010) *Clinical Judgement and Decision Making*. Maidenhead: Open University Press.

Standing, M (2014) *Clinical Judgement and Decision-Making for Nursing Students*, 2nd edn. London: SAGE Publications.

Stephenson, J (2014) *NHS England to Rollout '6Cs' Nursing Values to All Health Service Staff*. Nursing Times.net retrieved from www.nursingtimes.net/nursing-practice/specialisms/management/exclusive-6cs-nursing-values-to-be-rolled-out-to-all-nhs-staff/5070102.article

Stets, JE and Carter, MJ (2011) The moral self: applying identity theory. *Social Psychology Quarterly*, 74: 192–215.

Sully, P and Dallas, J (2005) *Essential Communication Skills for Nursing*. Edinburgh: Elsevier Mosby.

Taylor, J and Wros, P (2007) Concept mapping: a nursing model for care planning. *Journal of Nursing Education*, 46: 211–16.

References

Walshe, K and Shortell, SM (2004) When things go wrong: how healthcare organisations deal with major failures. *Health Affairs*, 23 (3): 103–11.

Waterlow, J (2008) *The Waterlow Score*. Available from: www.judy-waterlow.co.uk

Weir-Hughes, D (2007) Reviewing nursing diagnoses. *Nursing Management*, 14: 32–5.

Welton, JM and Halloran, EJ (2005) Nursing diagnoses, diagnosis-related group, and hospital outcomes. *Journal of Nursing Administration*, 35: 541–9.

West, L, Alheit, P, Anderson, AS et al. (eds) (2007) *Using Biographical and Life History Approaches in the Study of Adult and Lifelong Learning: European Perspectives*. Frankfurt am Main: Peter Lang.

Wilkinson, JM and Ahern, NR (2009) *Nursing Diagnosis Handbook*, 9th edn. Upper Saddle River, NJ: Prentice Hall.

Worden, A and Challis, D (2008) Care planning systems in care homes for older people. *Quality in Ageing*, 8: 28–38.

World Health Organization and United Nation's Children's Fund (1978) *Primary Health Care: Report of the International Conference on Primary Health Care*. Alma-Ata USSR. 26 September 1978. Geneva: WHO.

World Health Organization (2001) *Community Health Needs Assessment: An Introductory Guide for the Family Health Nurse in Europe*. Available from: www.euro.who.int/__data/assets/pdf_file/0018/102249/E73494.pdf

Index

6Cs 8–9, 17, 23, 95, 117, 157

accountability 147, 149, 152
accurate patient assessment 23–5
Acorns project 123
action planning 49; CHNA 131, 132
action research and clinical audit 27, 143, 148, 159
activities of daily living (ADLs) 93, 97–9, 103, 104, 106, 107, 127, 135
actual nursing diagnosis 74, 77
adaptation model 96–7, 103, 104, 106, 107
Aggleton, P. 102
Ahern, N.R. 66
Alma Ata declaration 128
ambulatory care settings 43
American Nurses Association 69
anaemia 160
analytical decision-making 144
analytical thinking 62
anxiety 83–4
archives 43
arteriogram 160
assessment tools 2, 24, 25, 51–64, 95; and audit 61; knowledge and skills needed 54–6; MUST 56–7, 63; NEWS 58–60, 63; potential problems 56; purpose 53–4; relationship to making a nursing diagnosis 60–1; Waterlow pressure ulcer scoring system 58, 63
Aston, L. 116, 117
attentive listening 14
audit 61, 63
autonomy 112, 113–14, 119

Barrett, D. 53, 71, 85
beliefs 11–12, 20
beneficence 112, 114–15
biographical details 37
body language 22, 160
body mass index (BMI) 56, 62

care 8, 9; organisational aspects of care ESC 51–2, 65–6, 78–9, 92–3, 109, 122, 138; philosophy of 112–13
care, compassion and communication ESC 6, 18–19, 33, 78, 92, 108–9, 122, 138
care pathways 95
care planning 2, 71–2, 78–91; connection between nursing therapy and nursing care outcomes 89–90; ethics and 112–16, 117; identifying a nursing problem 82–4; nursing models and decision-making in 103–4, 107; rationale for 80–2; stages 84–6, 87–8; written care plan 86–9
caring priorities 82
Carpenito-Moyet, L.J. 44, 66, 67, 71, 74–5
Carper, B. 22, 69
Chalmers, H. 102
choice 80, 81
clinical assessment skills 56, 62

clinical audits 61, 63; action research and clinical audit 27, 143, 148, 159
clinical decision-making *see* decision-making
clinical information 36
clinical judgement 2–3, 160; assessment, decision-making and healthcare interventions 139–43, 157–8; *see also* decision-making
closed questions 40, 41
cognitive continuum 3, 26–8, 143–4, 160; *see also* nine modes of practice
collaborative decision-making 146, 148, 151
collaborative working 52–3, 128–9, 129–30, 132, 142
commitment 8, 31
communication 8; care, compassion and communication ESC 6, 18–19, 33, 78, 92, 108–9, 122, 138; communication and interpersonal skills standard 5, 33, 108, 121, 137; skills 39–40, 82
community health needs assessment (CHNA) 2, 121–36; as an assessment process 127; five-step structured approach 131–3; importance of knowing about 126; nature of 124–6; preparation for 130–1; usefulness 127–9; who carries it out 129–30
community nurses 129, 130–1; origins of community nursing 123–4
community projects/initiatives 124, 126
compassion 8, 9, 31, 83–4; care, compassion and communication ESC 6, 18–19, 33, 78, 92, 108–9, 122, 138
compassion fatigue 9
competence 8, 31
concept mapping 90
confidence 147, 149, 152
confidentiality 116–17
consequentialism 110–11, 118
consultation exercise 128
coping mechanisms 44–5, 96–7
core values (6Cs) 8–9, 17, 23, 95, 117, 157
courage 8, 20
critical review of experiential and research evidence 27, 143, 159
critical thinking 103
Cruse 72, 160
culture 12, 16; ethical problems and 116–17; workplace 12–14, 16
Cummins, J. 8
CVA (cerebrovascular accident) 160

decision-making 2–3, 84, 137–59, 160; applying decision theory and research 143–4; assessment, clinical judgement, healthcare interventions and 139–43, 157–8; comparing nine modes of practice and ten perceptions 147–9; matrix model/ten perceptions 2–3, 146–52; nine modes of practice 3, 27–8, 31, 143–6, 158–9; nursing models and 103–4, 107; nursing practice and decision making standard 18, 33, 51, 65, 78, 92, 121, 137; 'PERSON' evaluation tool 3, 152–7, 160

Index

deficit view 35
delirium 160
demography 124
deontology 111, 118
Department of Health 126, 127–8
descriptive assessment tools 53
developmental stressors 100–1
diabetes 38, 115
diagnosis: assessment, clinical judgement, decision-making and healthcare interventions 139–43, 157–8; medical 67–8; nursing *see* nursing diagnosis
diagnostic cluster 75
discharge planning 81, 126, 135
disease distribution 133
district nurses 123, 134–5
documentation 24, 43, 71
Dougherty, L. 102

ECG (electrocardiogram) 160
Egan, G. 14, 39
Ellis, P. 40
epidemiology 124
epigastric pain 160
Essential Skills Clusters (ESCs) 3, 6, 18–19, 33, 51–2, 65–6, 78–9, 92–3, 108–9, 122, 138
ethical sensitivity 147, 148, 152
ethics 2, 108–20; ethical theories 110–12; problems with ethics as theory and ethics in practice 116–18; relevance of ethical theories to patient assessment and care planning 112–16
European Pressure Ulcer Advisory Panel classification system 61
evaluation 71; care planning 84, 85, 87–8; CHNA 131, 132; 'PERSON' evaluation tool 3, 152–7, 160
evidence 27–8
evidence-based care 153–7
experience and intuition decision-making 147, 148, 151
experimental research 27, 143, 159
explaining to the patient 55
exudate 60–1, 160

facts 25–7, 31
fairness 128
fibroadenoma 67, 160
flow chart 142
food kitchen project 130
Francis Report 9, 153
functional problems 44–5

Girard, N.J. 25
Glasgow Coma Scale 160
glucocorticoids 38, 160
glycohaemoglobin blood test 38
goal setting 71, 84, 85, 87–8, 91
Goodman, M. 22

Hall, A. 22
health inequalities, reducing 80, 90, 128
health needs assessment (HNA) 125, 126
health priorities 131, 132
health promotion 80, 112

health screening and diagnosis tools 53; *see also* assessment tools
health visitors 123, 135
healthcare failures 7
healthcare interventions *see* nursing/healthcare interventions
Hippocrates 112
holistic care 150–2
holistic perspective 35, 68
hypoglycaemia 66, 160

ice breakers 40
idiocultures 12, 160
implementation strategies 71, 72
in vitro fertilisation 112
incidence 132–3
inefficiency, reducing 80
information: for a CHNA 130, 132, 135–6; patient *see* patient information
informational needs 67
ingestion 160
Innes, A. 10
institutional differences 43
integrated care pathways 95
integrated healthcare teams 39, 128
interdependence 96–7, 105
interpersonal skills 5, 33, 108, 121, 137
interpretation 45–6, 49
interventions *see* nursing/healthcare interventions
intuitive judgement 27, 143, 144, 148, 158

justice 112, 115–16; social 128

Kitwood, T. 10
knowledge: factual 25–7; needed for using assessment tools 54–6; nursing 22

laddering questions 42
leadership, management and team working standard 18, 65, 78, 121, 137
leading questions 40
lifeworld 20–1
lines of resistance 101, 106
listening 8; attentive 14
Lister, S. 102
local planning 128
local policy 58

Maben, J. 10
MacPherson, S. 10
Malnutrition Universal Screening Tool (MUST) 56–7, 63
Manchester and Salford Ladies Sanitary Association 123
Manley, K. 12
matrix model 146–52; application to patient assessment, clinical decision-making and healthcare 149–52
McCabe, L. 10
McCance, T. 10, 11, 83
McCormack, B. 10, 11, 83
medical diagnosis 67–8

medical history 37, 75
medicine 35
memory 43
Mental Capacity Act (2005) 113, 119
mental health 35; problems 80–2
Mental Health Act (1983) amended (2007) 81
mindfulness 12, 160
modes of practice *see* nine modes of practice
Moule, P. 22
multiple questions 40
multi-professional/multi-agency working 128–9

National Early Warning Score (NEWS) 58–9, 63
National Institute for Health and Care Excellence (NICE) 54, 56, 59, 131
Neuman's system 100–1, 103, 104, 106, 107
neurology 160
neuropathy 160
NHS Plan 127–8
Nightingale, F. 68, 123
nine modes of practice 3, 27–8, 31, 143–6; application to patient assessment 144–6, 158–9; compared with ten perceptions of decision making 147–9
Nolan, D. 40
non-maleficence 112, 115
North American Nursing Diagnosis Association (NANDA) 69
nurse's priorities 127, 135
nurse's role in patient assessment 22–3
nursing diagnosis 2, 65–77; advantages and disadvantages 69–70; care planning 84, 85, 87–8; categories of 74–5; defining 66–8; developing from a patient assessment 74–6; history and development of 68–9; key aspects of 67; potential benefits and problems 72–4; relation to patient assessment process 70–2; relationship of screening tools to 60–1
nursing/healthcare interventions 93–4; assessment, clinical judgement, decision-making and 139–43, 157–8; care planning 84, 85, 87–8, 89, 91
nursing knowledge 22
Nursing and Midwifery Council (NMC): code of conduct 20, 31, 111, 118; Essential Skills Clusters (ESCs) 3, 6, 18–19, 33, 51–2, 65–6, 78–9, 92–3, 108–9, 122, 138; Standards for Pre-registration Nursing Education 3, 5, 18, 33, 51, 65, 78, 92, 108, 121, 137
nursing and midwifery strengths and weaknesses 153–7
nursing models 2, 92–107; framing the assessment process 102–3, 106–7; impacting on decision-making in care planning 103–4, 107; importance 94–5; Neuman's system 100–1, 103, 104, 106, 107; Orem's self-care model 99–100, 103, 104, 106, 107; Roper, Logan and Tierney's activities of daily living 93, 97–9, 103, 104, 106, 107, 127, 135; Roy's adaptation model 96–7, 103, 104, 106, 107; skills needed by the practitioner 95, 105
nursing practice and decision making standard 18, 33, 51, 65, 78, 92, 121, 137
nursing priorities 43–5, 49, 127–8, 135

nursing problems, identifying 82–4, 85, 87–8
nursing process 69, 70–3, 95
nutrition and fluid management ESC 52

objective information 24, 35–8
objectivity 24
observation 36, 37; decision-making based on 146, 148, 151
occupational therapy 35
oesophageal gastroduodenoscopy 160
open questions 40, 41
Orem's self-care model 99–100, 103, 104, 106, 107
organisational aspects of care ESC 51–2, 65–6, 78–9, 92–3, 109, 122, 138
outcomes: connection between nursing therapy and 89–90; evaluation of 71, 84, 85, 87–8; outcomes of care benefit the patient in 'PERSON' 153–7

patient assessment 1, 18–32; applying the matrix model 149–52; clinical judgement, decision-making and healthcare interventions 139–43, 157–8; dealing with facts 25–7; defining 20–1; developing a nursing diagnosis from 74–6; framing using a nursing model 102–3, 106–7; importance of accuracy 23–5; nature of truth 28–9; nine modes of practice applied to 143–6, 158–9; nurse's role 22–3; person-centred 21; 'PERSON' evaluation tool 152–7; relationship of nursing diagnosis to 70–2; relevance of ethical theories to 112–16; Standing's cognitive continuum 27–8; stereotyping 29–30
patient-centredness 153–7; *see also* person-centredness
patient information 1–2, 33–50, 75; analysing and identifying nursing priorities 43–5, 49; defining 35; problems in information gathering 43; questioning techniques 39–43, 48–9; sense-making and interpreting to others 45–6, 49; types and forms of information 35–8; when to assess patients 38–9, 48
patient involvement 45, 62, 82
patient and peer-aided judgement 27, 143, 148, 158
patient preferences 82
patient priorities 44, 45, 82, 127–8, 135
perceptions of decision-making *see* ten perceptions of decision-making
person-centred care 10–11, 45, 150–2
Person-Centred Health and Care Collaborative 9
person-centredness 1, 5–17, 83, 91; core values 8–9, 17, 23, 95, 117, 157; defining 9–11; values and beliefs 11–12, 20; ways of working 14–15; workplace culture 12–14, 16
'PERSON' evaluation tool 3, 152–7, 160
personal feelings 22–3, 111, 118
personalised care 80, 81
personhood 9–10
philosophy of care 112–13
physiology 96–7, 105; stressors 100–1
population, identifying 131
possible diagnosis 74
potential problems, risk-assessing 115
predictive assessment tools 53

Index

prescription 37
pressure sore prevalence audits 61
prevalence 132–3
Price, B. 42
priorities 23; analysing patient information 43–5, 49; CHNA 131, 132; differences in priorities between patients and healthcare professionals 127, 135; nursing priorities 43–5, 49, 127–8, 135; patient priorities 44, 45, 82, 127–8, 135; prioritising decision-making 147, 148, 151
probing questions 40, 41
problem identification 82–4, 85, 87-8
PRODUCT criterion 85
professional experience 43
professional values standard 5, 18, 108, 121, 137
prognosis 161
prompt cues 42
psychological stressors 100–1
public health 122–3, 125; *see also* community health needs assessment (CHNA)
public opinion 127–8

qualitative research 27, 143, 159
quality improvement agenda 7–9
questioning techniques 39–43, 48–9

record keeping 43
referral information 37
reflection 47, 69, 73
reflective decision-making 147, 148, 151
reflective judgement 27, 143, 148, 158
repeated information 36
resourcing issues 80, 115–16
review 131, 132
review dates 84, 86, 87–8
rhetorical questions 40
risk assessment 112, 115; risks assessed and managed 153–7
risk diagnosis 74, 77
risk factors 44
Rogers, C. 9
role functions 96–7
Roper, Logan and Tierney's activities of daily living 93, 97–9, 103, 104, 106, 107, 127, 135
Royal College of Nursing (RCN) 22, 125, 130–1
Roy's adaptation model 96–7, 103, 104, 106, 107

safe and effective delivery of care 153–7
Scotland 9; community initiative 124
screening tools *see* assessment tools
self-care model 99–100, 103, 104, 106, 107
self-concept 96–7, 105
sense-making 45–6, 49
sensual information 36
6Cs 8–9, 17, 23, 95, 117, 157
SMART goals 85
social context 37
social justice 128
social work 35
sociocultural stressors 100–1
solution-focused working 14–15, 17

spiritual needs 73–4, 77
spiritual stressors 100–1
standardisation of terms 66–8
standardised decision-making 146, 148, 151
Standards for Pre-registration Nursing Education 3, 5, 18, 33, 51, 65, 78, 92, 108, 121, 137
Standing, M. 153; cognitive continuum (nine modes of practice) 3, 26–8, 143–4; ten perceptions of decision-making 2–3, 146–7
stent 59, 161
stereotyping 29–30
strategic planning 71
strategy implementation 71
strengths 14–15, 44; nursing and midwifery strengths and weaknesses 153–7
stressors 100–1, 106
subjective information 24, 35–8
subjectivity 24; truth and 28–9
survey research 27, 143, 159
sympathetic presence 82, 83–4, 89
symptoms 37
syndrome diagnosis 75, 77
system-aided judgement 27, 143, 148, 159
systematic decision-making 146, 148, 151
systematic thinking 71–3

targeting services/resources 128
technology 43
ten perceptions of decision making 2–3, 146–52; compared with nine modes of practice 147–9; *see also* matrix model
terminology 66
test results 37
therapeutic relationship 82, 83–4, 89–90
think-aloud reasoning process 83
timing of patient assessment 38–9, 48
Treehouse food kitchen project 130
truth 28–9

ulcerative colitis 57, 161
unexplained weight loss 56–7, 62–3
United States of America (USA) 69
upstreaming 130–1
urisheath 114, 161

values 11–12, 20; core (6Cs) 8–9, 17, 23, 95, 117, 157; professional values standard 5, 18, 108, 121, 137
visualisation distraction 84

Waterlow pressure ulcer scoring system 58, 63
ways of working, person-centred 14–15
weight loss, unexplained 56–7, 62–3
wellness 75
Wilkinson, J.M. 66
Williamson, L. 130
workplace culture 12–14, 16
wound assessment 24, 25; charts 25, 60
written care plan 86–9

Your Health, Your Care, Your Say 128